food allergy & your child

a practical guide for parents

Alice Willitts and Deborah Carter

Mothers of anaphylactic children.

Medical Adviser: Professor John O. Warner MD FRCPCH FMed Sci

Professor of Paediatrics, Imperial College, St Mary's Campus, London since September 2006. Previously Professor of Child Health at the University of Southampton where he ran a large paediatric allergy clinic. He has been involved with paediatric allergy and respiratory research for 30 years and written over 300 articles on paediatric allergy and respiratory topics. He is Editor-in-Chief of Paediatric Allergy and Immunology and he runs the paediatric allergy clinic at St Mary's Hospital, London.

Dietitian: Kate Grimshaw BSc MSc SRD RNutr

Research Dietitian for the University of Southampton specialising in food allergy. Currently working on a Food Standards Agency study looking at the relationship between infant feeding in the first year and allergy development. This study forms part of a pan-European study. She is a member of the Food Allergy and Intolerance specialist group of the British Dietetic Association and is co-ordinator for the food allergy module of the MSc in Allergy run at Southampton University. She provides dietetic advice for the acute allergy clinic for families at Southampton General Hospital.

The authors welcome feedback from the readers of this work:
authors@allergychild.org.uk

First published 2007
Class Publishing, Barb House, Barb Mews, London W6 7PA, UK
Telephone: (020) 7371 2119
Fax: (020) 7371 2878
Email: post@class.co.uk
Website: www.class.co.uk

A CIP catalogue record for this book is available from the British Library.

ISBN 9781859591864

Design: Simon Blacker, Blacker Design
Illustration: Eve Peasnall

Printed in China by 1010 Printing

Contents

Forewords

I am delighted to have the opportunity to write a foreword to this outstanding practical book on food allergy and your child.

All allergic problems, including food allergy, have increased significantly in prevalence in developed countries around the world over the last 30 to 40 years. While we have some ideas about why this increase has occurred, sadly we are not yet able to either prevent allergy occurring in the first place or cure it. I obviously hope and expect that research will identify strategies that will change this in the future. However, for the present it is most important that your child has an accurate allergy diagnosis and that you are given appropriate advice on how to handle it. This is no easy matter, and having practical advice from 'the horse's mouth' will be invaluable in your quest for help. Deborah Carter and Alice Willitts have personal experience of the trials and tribulations of working through the health system and coming to terms with the problem. They have also sought input from other families and have been able to produce an invaluable source of very important and useful information.

Having a child with a food allergy has a great impact on quality of life, creating enormous and understandable anxieties for the present and future. However, it is possible to gain a realistic acceptance of the problem and to carry on enjoying life to the full. Deborah and Alice have shown, through their own experiences, that this is possible.

I not only feel that this book will be of value to parents of children with food allergy but also to health professionals. They would do well to read it very carefully to help give them insights into all the issues and problems that are faced by families once food allergy has been diagnosed. This will facilitate a shared understanding of the problem and a vision of how it should be handled in the future.

Professor John O. Warner MD FRCPCH FMed Sci
Professor of Paediatrics, Imperial College, St Mary's Campus, London.

Food allergy can be worrying, there's no doubt about that. The thousands of callers who contact our helpline each year will testify to that. But the risks are most certainly manageable. Families affected can learn how to raise their children in an atmosphere of safety and stability.

Those were core messages of the Anaphylaxis Campaign when the charity was founded in early 1994, and I firmly believe that they still hold true today.

However, something is often lacking to help families achieve a well-balanced approach. People need high-quality, reliable help and information, and such support is sometimes hard to come by. Allergy services in many parts of the country are inadequate. GPs sometimes struggle to point the patient in the right direction. There is information available on the Internet, but much of it is of questionable worth.

That is why this extremely helpful and comprehensive book will prove so valuable to any parent of a child with food allergy. It offers insights that the authors are well placed to give – having 'been there' themselves.

Our charity is at the forefront of the food allergy debate and we know how common it is for misinformation to affect people's judgement. But Alice Willitts and Deborah Carter have approached the problems from a very well-informed and pragmatic standpoint and have avoided many of the pitfalls that some magazine and newspaper writers fall into.

For more than a decade, I have been meeting families who tell me they find coping with food allergy a nightmare. That is completely understandable. The problems associated with food labelling, eating out, and children's parties may seem overwhelming. I am sure if those families had had this book to guide them, life wouldn't have seemed anywhere near so hard.

David Reading OBE
Director, the Anaphylaxis Campaign

Acknowledgements

We would like to thank all those who have helped us with the production of this book, giving their time and expertise generously, especially: John Warner for his supervision, guidance and enthusiastic support, Kate Grimshaw for opening our eyes with her liberated approach to feeding allergic children, David Reading for his advice and guidance, John de Mora for his belief in our project, Eve Peasnall for her delightful pictures, and Simon Blacker and Anne Willitts for their invaluable help in turning our text into a book.

We would also like to thank all the parents and children who gave their personal stories to this book to help others face the day-to-day challenges of bringing up allergic children.

Special thanks go to Lincoln Medical whose generous funding enabled us to produce the book, our way.

Alice and Deborah

Thanks to the friends who looked after my children so lovingly while I wrote, especially Helen, Ali, Julia, Jenny and Lucy; to all our kind Allergy Buddies; to my parents John and Claire, thank you for your tireless support with childcare and in editing this text; to my husband Martin for his unwavering encouragement and conviction that writing this book was valuable and last but not least, to Zac with whom I've learnt so much and for being just wonderful.

Alice

I wish to thank everybody who helped me to care for Thomas in those early days and bring him to full health especially Angela Meyrick-Jones (Health Visitor), Julia Milligan (GP) and the staff at Southampton General Hospital. I want to tell Thomas I feel privileged to be his mum and thank him for his resilience throughout. I wish also to thank my daughters Rachel, Sarah and Isabel for their care and patience when his needs were placed before theirs. The writing of this book is testimony to the bravery of the children affected by allergy and to the dedication and love given them by their parents.

Deborah

Introduction

Food allergy amongst children is on the increase and if you are reading this book, the chances are you have a child who is being made ill by the food he or she eats. Whether the cause is intolerance or allergy it is distressing to see your child suffer as a result of eating everyday foods.

This book offers parents and carers of children with food allergies a practical guide to dealing successfully with the real, everyday situations you'll find yourself facing.

You may, especially in the early days, wonder whether you can manage a special diet, keep your child safe, or even get him or her to adulthood. By passing on the experiences of other parents, we aim to guide you through the incredibly difficult first months when all the information coming at you is new and the lifestyle you were used to is changing fast.

When our own children were first diagnosed we searched for guidance on how to manage everyday living and found none. The information available was largely geared towards allergic adults and came from medical experts. It seemed to us that unless you happened to know someone who had a severely allergic child, you were on a lonely path without a map or compass.

Having friends who share an understanding of what you're going through, be it sleepless nights, weaning, potty training or wobbles about a first day at school, is comforting and reassuring. Suddenly we found our friends could not share these new fears and worries with us and even meeting up for a play-date became stressful. Doctors couldn't answer our questions either as parenting food allergic children is not their area of expertise.

Trawling through bookshops, libraries and the internet we found no books that charted the emotional territory of bringing up a food-allergic child. None held the stories and insights of others who'd been there before. We felt that it was time the experiences were passed on, not lost only to be learnt afresh by each new parent facing this turmoil. We sought out other allergic families and it quickly became apparent that we were not the only ones who would appreciate a more anecdotal guide to food allergy.

We interviewed and talked to many families with different experiences of living with food allergy. Some were positive, some negative; some had good support networks, some had none; some had money to throw at the problem, others were wholly reliant on the NHS and state provision for care and support. We also talked to those who had severe, multiple allergies often compounded by asthma or eczema; others who had milder allergies to perhaps only one foodstuff. We gathered together all these fragments of information and started piecing together what eventually became this book.

We have chosen to present our research in a loosely chronological structure reflecting the order in which most parents face issues, starting with the fast-track pages containing the information you will need at diagnosis. Later chapters explore the practicalities and emotional upheaval having an allergic child brings. We look at key moments in your child's life that are made harder by their food allergy such as finding childcare, going on holiday, birthday parties and starting school.

It is clear that there is no right or wrong way to react to the diagnosis of a life-threatening condition in your child. We all respond according to our personality and circumstances coupled with our expectations of parenthood. Personal and professional situations play a part, as do pressures from family and friends, society and the medical professionals in whose care we find ourselves.

Although we conceived this book in 2002, writing about food allergy is still largely the province of medical experts as we take the book to print in 2007. We have been fortunate enough to have the invaluable guidance of specialists Professor John O. Warner and Kate Grimshaw who have addressed all the medical and dietary questions we could not have answered.

We are not specialists, just women who have been through the experience of living with severely allergic children and feel passionately that those best placed to inform other parents facing the same challenges are those who've actually been there. If this book helps just one other family come to terms with this life-changing experience then it will have been worth all the effort.

We wish you all the best.
Alice and Deborah

Fast-track information

Our aim in this section is to help fast-track you to the best allergy information and support available. From our own experience and that of our interviewees, we know that you will need information and support from a variety of sources. We also know how hard it is to access reliable help quickly. The tried and tested pointers here will provide you with a reference framework which you can source yourself, from home, from bookshops or libraries, and digest at your own speed.

Where to start

The first few days after your child has had an allergic reaction can be a bewildering and frightening time. Although you may have heard that allergies to food are on the increase, the discovery that your own child is affected can still come as a dreadful shock. Your easy, confident approach to food is brought abruptly to an end. You can no longer simply *feed* your child, instead a laborious process of vetting every scrap of food is about to begin. At the moment, the future may seem daunting but do not despair. Over time, you will find that it is possible to build a relaxed, natural relationship with food again.

So what do you do first? Who can you turn to? What kind of help do you need most?

Information about your child's allergy

- Ring Allergy UK (01322 619898) and ask for advice and fact sheets or talk to an allergy nurse. This Helpline is open 9am–5pm, Monday to Friday. You can request up to five fact sheets online at www.allergyuk.org which will be emailed directly to you. You can also order by telephone (01322 619898) or by post from Allergy UK, 3 White Oak Square, Swanley, Kent BR8 7AG.

  Allergy UK is a national medical charity established to increase understanding and awareness of allergy, to help people manage their allergies, to raise funds for allergy research and to provide training in allergy for healthcare professionals including doctors, nurses, dietitians and pharmacists.[1]

- Ring the Anaphylaxis Campaign (01252 542029) and ask for advice and fact sheets. This Helpline is open 9am-5pm, Monday to Friday. There is an answerphone service at other times. You can request fact sheets by email at: info@anaphylaxis.org.uk or via the website at www.anaphylaxis.org.uk

  The Anaphylaxis Campaign is a membership-based organisation which provides information and guidance, primarily to its members and to potential members, but also to the media, health professionals and food companies. There is also a strong campaigning role, particularly in the areas of product labelling and allergy services. The Campaign has a range of educational products including information sheets, videos and a children's book.[2]

- Ring your health visitor and ask her to come to the house. Talk to her at length. Health visitors are trained listeners and can offer non-judgemental support. She may be able to tell you whether there is a doctor in your practice who has a particular interest in allergy or if there is a local allergy support group.

Life with an allergic child is not as bad as we first feared but it is frustrating.
Angela

To talk to someone who's been there

- Allergy UK (01322 619898) has a Support Contact list. Ask them to put you in touch with another parent of an allergic child to whom you can talk by telephone.
- Have the courage to actually phone the Support Contact! Sharing your experience can be invaluable.
- Phone the Anaphylaxis Campaign Helpline (01252 542029) to talk to an allergy advisor and find out about the local support groups they run nationally.
- Your health visitor may be able to put you in touch with local parents of allergic children.

I deal with stress at the time but afterwards realise how much it's taken out of me. Then I don't want to think about it, I just feel glad it's over. At the time, I probably didn't ask for help loudly enough. I was just coming to terms with having a baby you've got to care for anyway and then leaving her to go back to work. There was just too much going on, it was the last thing I needed, to be honest. Alison

Some breathing space

- Ask a close friend or relative to come round for a few hours or even stay with you for a few days. You will then be free to concentrate on preparing appropriate meals for your child and also to do some reading and thinking.
- Could your partner take a day off work?
- Ask your health visitor about arranging help in the home through an agency such as Home Start (www.home-start.org.uk or 08000 686368).
- Be prepared to let everything else slide for a while. There isn't much in life that can't be put on hold, cancelled or passed onto a helpful friend.
- You may find you benefit from some time off work to learn about caring for your allergic child and to pass on this new information to your childminder or the nursery (pp.127, 137). You are legally entitled to unpaid parental leave by agreement with your employer, if you can afford to take it.
- Put your baby in the pushchair and go for a walk. This is a great way to think. Take a pen and paper and jot down your thoughts.
- Find someone you can talk to who is concerned with your emotional needs, not just the practical stuff.
- Have a good cry!

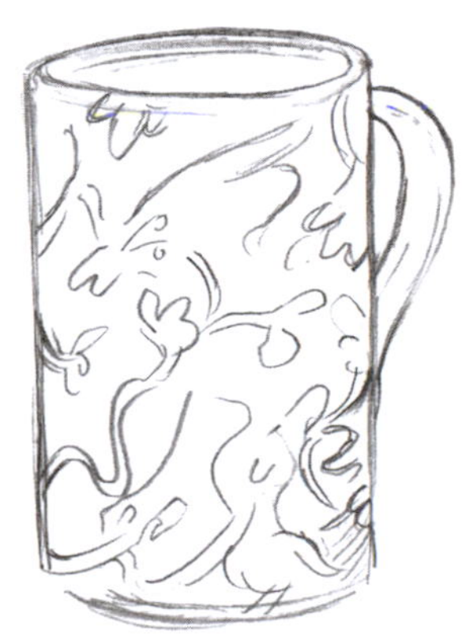

Help with what to feed your child

- Read *Let's get practical* p.62 for a guide to weaning, shopping and cooking.
- Send for a 'Free From...' list from your local supermarket (p.82). Telephone numbers are listed in the Appendix.
- Ask your GP to refer you to a dietitian, who will help you devise a menu and work out which foods to introduce and when. If you would like to see a dietitian quickly, discuss with your GP the possibility of a private appointment.

Books on allergy

Many books have been written explaining why and how allergies affect us. The books listed here represent the ones we have found most useful. Together they will give you a thorough understanding of allergy; individually they have particular strengths which we highlight below.

The Allergy Bible by **Linda Gamlin**, ISBN: 978-1844001729
A comprehensive guide to allergies. Clearly written and illustrated, this will give you a sound understanding of current medical knowledge and why allergies affect the people they do. You'll dip into this again and again.

The Complete Guide to Food Allergy and Intolerance by **Prof. Jonathan Brostoff & Linda Gamlin**, ISBN: 978-0747534303
A more in-depth examination of the mechanism of allergy accompanied by case histories. Has useful chapters specific to allergies in children, also a detailed breakdown of food groups and potential cross reactions.

Food Allergies – enjoying life with a severe food allergy by **Tanya Wright**, ISBN: 185959039X or Second Edition: 978-1859591468
A superb, practical guide for adults with severe food allergies – many of the same rules apply for children. Detailed information on manufacturers and stockists of allergy-friendly products.

Allergies at Your Fingertips by **Dr Joanne Clough**, ISBN: 9781872362526
In a question and answer format, this book addresses 312 real questions from people with allergies. First published in 1998 it is still useful today and revised editions are available.

My advice: read everything you can about it. Then you can feel a bit more confident about your decisions. I wish I'd known that experts' opinions vary, sometimes quite a lot. You want guidance but at the end of the day, they're giving you an opinion and you're the one who has to weigh that up against others. You get to that stage where you've immersed yourself in it and can feel you've made a good decision but it's time consuming. Gwyneth

Allergy websites

The beauty of the web is its immediacy. You can access it at any hour of the day or night for a global perspective on any issue. One disadvantage can be that it throws up so much information that it is sometimes hard to pick what is most relevant. The websites listed here will provide you with accurate information on your child's particular allergies and links to other useful sites. We have chosen them because they are the sites most relevant to *children* with allergies and are, quite simply, the best of the bunch.

www.anaphylaxis.org: Canadian Anaphylaxis site. A positive, practical guide to anaphylaxis which aims to help the whole family. Features real-life accounts and a 'Safe4Kids' page where allergic children share experiences and can learn by themselves.

www.allergyfacts.org.au: A great Australian site specialising in children's allergies which provides factual and practical information for parents. Features cartoon characters who suffer from various allergies to help young children understand. Older children can send messages, poems and pictures to others with similar experiences.

www.allergicchild.com: An empathetic American site by the parents of two severely allergic children offering understanding along with practical information. Includes other parents' allergy stories and shared experiences.

www.anaphylaxis.org.uk: The Anaphylaxis Campaign website has a wealth of information about food allergies, particularly peanut allergy. The site also gives allergy guidance for pre-schools and schools.

www.allergyuk.org: The Allergy UK website. The site includes a list of the fact sheets available on request, product updates, information and advice on allergies in general.

Public libraries provide cheap access to the web if you do not have a computer at home.

Take heart

We know that you may well be feeling tired and emotional already as you begin to try and understand the implications of your child's allergies. You will meet your first hurdle with the very next meal and, as we all know, those mealtimes come round pretty fast with little time for contemplation in between. It is unlikely that you have had a full diagnosis of your child's allergens at this stage and you may be dealing with questions from friends and relatives that you are not yet equipped to answer.

It can feel as though your life has become dominated by your child's allergies and all you seem to be doing is reading, telephoning and writing to gather as much information as you can. Take heart, life will settle down again as you become more expert.

All this new information will almost certainly throw up questions and worries that you would like addressed. This book will answer many of them for you, but do make use of the health professionals available and the support contacts from allergy charities.

Glossary

Here we explain what some of the words associated with allergy that you will come across in this book mean. Also see *Medical terminology explained* (p.30).

adrenaline a hormone produced naturally in the human body. *Epinephrine* is the name given to the manufactured substance found in adrenaline auto-injectors. When administered in an *anaphylactic reaction, epinephrine* reverses the symptoms by acting on the body in the same way as natural adrenaline – it normalises blood pressure and circulation.

adrenaline auto-injector a spring-activated auto-injector containing a sterile, single dose of adrenaline. Anapen® and EpiPen® are the registered trademarks for brands referred to in this book. Also called adrenaline pens or injector pens.

allergen/allergenic a substance that can trigger an *allergic reaction*.

allergenic foods in *children* the most common allergens are cow's milk, eggs, peanuts, tree nuts (almonds, hazelnuts, walnuts, cashews, pecans, Brazils, pistachios, macadamia nuts and Queensland nuts), fish, shellfish, soya and wheat which make up 98 per cent of all childhood allergens.

allergic reaction a reaction that occurs when the body's *immune system* encounters an *allergen* and produces *antibodies* called *immunoglobulin E* (*IgE antibodies*) which trigger the *mast cells* to release chemicals into the body.

allergy/allergies an abnormal or inappropriate reaction of the body's *immune system* to a substance (an *allergen*) that would normally be harmless.

allergy-friendly someone or something that reduces the risk of exposure to *allergens*.

anaphylaxis/anaphylactic/anaphylactic reaction/anaphylactic shock a sudden, severe *allergic reaction* to an *allergen* that can be life-threatening.

antibody/antibodies produced by the *immune system* in response to a foreign substance, *antibodies* circulate in the blood serum. Their purpose is to help to fight infection and foreign elements (eg. bacteria, parasites).

antihistamines drugs that block the action of *histamine*.

asthma a lung disease in which inflammation of the airways and spasms of the airway wall muscles make it difficult to move air in and out of the lungs causing wheezing, coughing and tightness of the chest making it difficult to breathe.

atopic/atopy a genetic (inherited) tendency to develop an *allergy* or *allergies*.

cross-contamination comes from mixing unsafe foods with safe ones by using the same utensils, pans, crockery or chopping boards. (See also pp.88, 110)

dairy/dairy products cow's milk, or products made from cow's milk.

diagnostic used to assist diagnosis (eg allergic history, allergy tests).

eczema an inflammatory condition of the skin that makes the skin itch. Skin can appear dry and scaly but it can become red, blistered and weepy.

epinephrine the name used worldwide for the manufactured *adrenaline* found in adrenaline auto-injectors. When administered in an *anaphylactic reaction* epinephrine reverses the symptoms by acting on the body in the same way as *adrenaline* – it normalises blood pressure and circulation. In the UK, you will often still see *adrenaline* and *epinephrine* used in conjunction. We use the term adrenaline in this book.

food challenge a test that involves a substance, such as a suspected food, being given in increasing amounts to see if an *allergic reaction* will occur.

histamine a chemical produced naturally by the body and released in unusually high doses during an *allergic reaction* causing the symptoms of *allergy*.

hives another name for *urticaria*, also called nettle rash.

hydrolysate a formula milk containing modified milk protein that has significantly reduced allergic potential.

IgE / immunoglobulin E an *antibody* that is involved in *allergy* and *anaphylaxis*.

immune system the body's way of resisting external factors to protect itself. In *allergic* people the immune system over-reacts to substances (*allergens*) that are harmless in non-allergic people.

intolerance when the body reacts badly to a particular substance but without producing *IgE antibodies*; a reaction that does not involve the *immune system*.

mast cells are cells in the body which release chemicals (including *histamine*) into the body during an *allergic reaction*.

multiple allergies reacting to more than one substance (*allergen*).

nebuliser a piece of equipment used to administer drugs orally, to treat *asthma*.

nutrient a substance found in foods which provides essential nourishment.

phyto-oestrogen an oestrogen derived from a plant (eg soya). Oestrogen is a hormone that develops and maintains female characteristics in the human body.

RAST (radio-allergosorbent test) a *diagnostic* blood test for detecting *IgE antibodies* produced by the *immune system*, used to identify which *allergens* someone is *allergic* to.

skin-prick test *diagnostic* test used to identify which *allergens* someone is *allergic* to. Pricking gently through a drop of allergen extract placed on the arm may produce a small *weal* which indicates the presence of an *allergy*. The procedure is painless, gives rapid results and is probably the most commonly used *allergy* test.

steroids common abbreviation for corticosteroids, used to treat inflammation caused by allergy, usually administered in the form of drops, sprays, inhalers or creams and ointments.

urticaria itchy rash on the skin with *weals*, looks like nettle stings. Also called *hives* or nettle rash.

Ventolin a brand of inhaler used in the treatment of asthma.

weal a swelling on the skin, like a bump (as in *urticaria* or after *skin-prick testing*).

IN THE BEGINNING

1 Health professionals

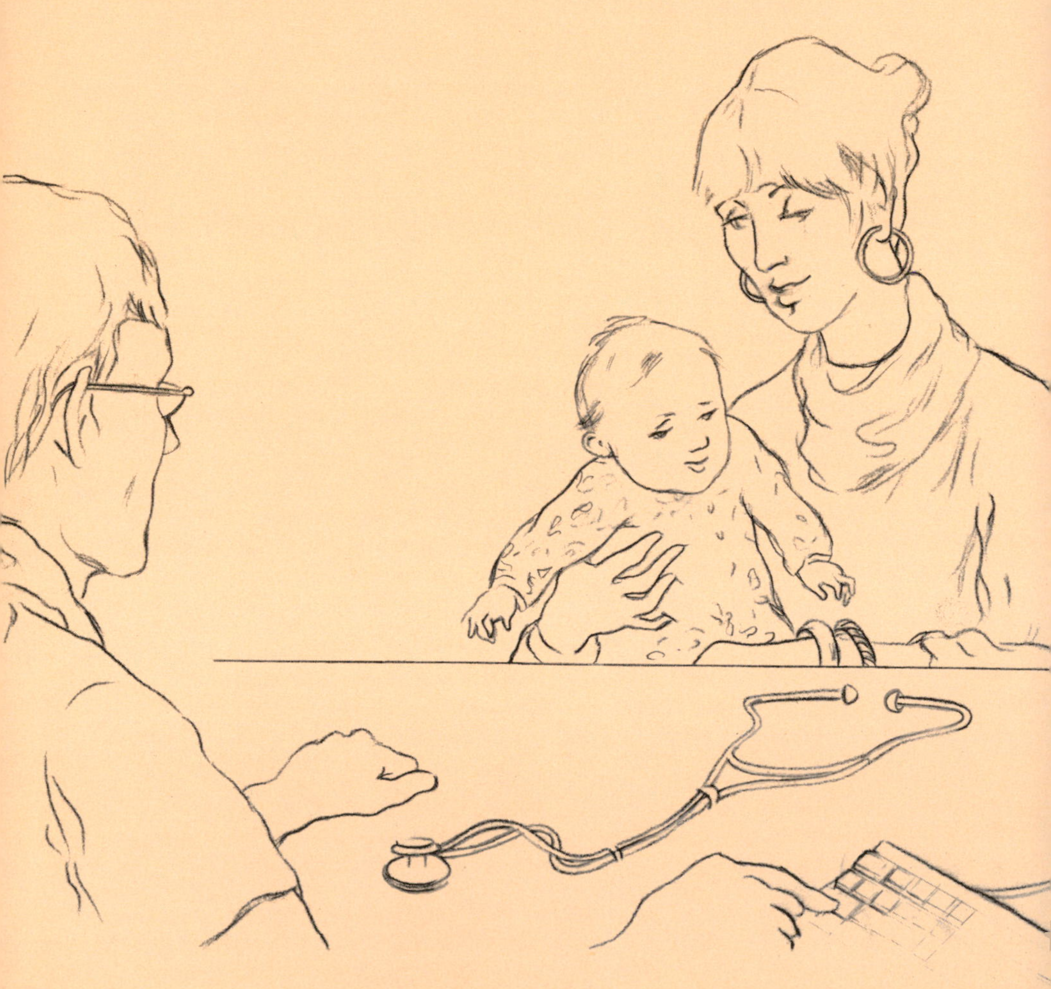

Whatever your route to diagnosis and treatment, here we offer guidance on what to expect from the range of health professionals you will meet along the way.

General Practitioners (GPs)

GPs are often the first people we see as frightened and anxious parents, and they may not live up to our expectations. GPs often receive a bad press from allergy parents (not all of it unfounded!). The problem appears to be that many GPs are not trained to deal with clinical allergy because the recent increase in allergic cases has rather caught the medical profession unawares.

Being realistic about the kind of help your GP can give you should help you get the most out of appointments. He or she can give you general medical advice and prescribe drugs including antihistamines, adrenaline and asthma and eczema medications. GPs can also refer your child to a paediatrician, allergist, dietitian or counsellor for specialist help. What they are not able to do is give you all the emotional support you need, or help you to plan an appropriate diet for your child.

A good relationship with your GP and continued support in managing your child's allergies is the ideal. If you feel you are not getting this support, it's worth considering the following:

Time pressure

The short time allocated for your doctor's appointment will go by incredibly fast so write down what you have to say and any questions you want to ask. If you need longer, it is quite okay to book a double appointment.

Your relationship with your doctor

What parents of allergic children need is a doctor who listens to their experience, takes their concerns seriously and helps them to find the best treatment as quickly as possible. Most doctors are aiming for this too. However, misunderstandings can arise on both sides because a doctor will examine your child with a professional detachment which, by its very nature, is different from your own deep, emotional involvement.

If, despite taking all that into account, you feel the doctor is not taking you seriously, take a deep breath and state your case clearly again. Try not to get agitated. The doctor may not appreciate the fear, frustration and anxiety that you are feeling and how this affects your ability to communicate. Bear in mind that not all doctors have actually witnessed an anaphylactic reaction, let alone had first-hand experience of parenting an allergic child. This does not of course mean that they cannot be sympathetic to your situation. They *can* help you.

Over the coming months and years you will need the support of your GP so it is worth building a good relationship. If you are continually battling with your doctor, find another you can relate to *and do it now*. If you can't find one in whom you have confidence, transfer to another local surgery. You can also talk the situation over with your health visitor who may be able to suggest a doctor with better allergy awareness. There are many fantastic GPs who do all they can for their allergy patients.

Our GP was superb, immediately recognising that the symptoms I was describing were the result of a mild allergy to milk. The doctor arranged for allergy testing at the hospital which was carried out before Peter was a year old. All along the doctors at our surgery have been sympathetic and aware of potential problems. Angela

Many parents will find that their doctor takes food allergy seriously, is sympathetic and thoroughly up to date. However, there are still doctors who are sceptical about the whole issue.

There's one doctor at our practice who I won't see any more. When Daisy had the first reaction to peanuts, I drove to the surgery first because I didn't know what to do. He could see she was having trouble breathing and said, 'There's not a lot we can do about it – she'll get over it.' But driving back I knew I wasn't happy so we went to the hospital. The nurse said, 'If they're wheezing and their lips are swelling, it's serious – don't mess about – call an ambulance.' She took it seriously. My instinct was right, the doctor was wrong, and that was important. I think that sort of blasé attitude is unforgivable. You know when there's something wrong with your child. Don't go against your own instincts. Alison

If you have any concerns about the advice from your GP, trust your instincts. Seek a second opinion by making an appointment to see another doctor in the practice and consult Allergy UK, the Anaphylaxis Campaign or NHS Direct to talk it over with people who know about allergy.

Dr Julia Milligan, a GP, describes her role in diagnosing and treating allergy:

- To listen to the patient. In the case of allergic children, I would expect the parents to tell me as much as they can.
- To try and determine what has caused the allergic reaction.
- To consider referring the patient for specific advice to an allergy clinic.
- To educate the parents and the patient on the prevention of contact with the allergen and appropriate treatment of future episodes.
- To give the patient relevant treatment such as antihistamines, adrenaline injection and salbutamol/steroids if appropriate. Give advice on calling the paramedics if the adrenaline injection needs to be given.
- To advise parents to ensure that carers, nursery and school staff are aware of the potential problem and have an appropriate management plan.

Asking questions

You may come away after the initial diagnosis relieved to know what is wrong with your child but, at the same time, in a state of shock. It is not until you are home that the reality of what you are facing sinks in and you may well feel that you haven't asked the right questions. You will almost certainly want to go back to your doctor to ask more questions.

Depression

It is all too easy to forget about your own health when you are concentrating all your energies on your child. Stress can lead to depression. Tell your GP if you are experiencing any of the following: feeling tired but unable to sleep; having no appetite or overeating; experiencing a loss of interest in yourself; finding the smallest chores too much to manage; feeling tearful, isolated or lonely; experiencing chronic anxiety, irritability or irrationality.

If you and your child share the same GP make consecutive appointments, one for you and one for your child, so that both sets of notes are available.

Try to be realistic about what the GP can do for you. He or she can prescribe antidepressants and/or refer you to a psychiatric nurse or sometimes directly to a counsellor. If you suspect that you are depressed, think about what sort of treatment you feel would suit you and discuss it with your GP. Also, see p.50 on emotional impact.

Health visitors

Health visitors can be a great source of support and help. Our advice is to make contact with your health visitor as soon as possible. She can:

- Visit you at home.
- Tell you where your nearest casualty department is.
- Help you find a sympathetic doctor.
- Reassure you that your child is developing normally.
- Help arrange for a 'mother's help' from an agency or local church group.
- Put you in touch with other parents of allergic children locally.
- Listen to you when you simply need to talk.
- Arrange for adrenaline auto-injector training in nurseries and schools (p.136).

My health visitor had a very common-sense attitude to our children and their health. She took an interest and just being able to talk to her was great. Gwyneth

Should your health visitor prove to be unsupportive, don't be afraid to ask to be transferred to another member of staff.

Health visitor Ellie Cross describes the help she can offer families with allergic children:

The best way your health visitor can help you through 'allergy hell' is by listening to and supporting both you and your family, before, during and after diagnosis. We have basic counselling skills to help you and your family discover solutions and come to terms with the challenges that lie ahead.

We are usually available for home visits, telephone and surgery consultations and often run drop-in clinics. Hopefully, you and your health visitor can design a package of care to meet the needs of you and your family. For example, it is often important to consider other siblings who may be indirectly affected by an allergy in the family and offer them a chance to be heard and supported too. We can also put you in contact with other local families in similar circumstances.

From a more practical point of view we can tell you about the professionals and experts who will be able to help and support you on your journey. We have access to psychologists, dietitians, school nurses, paediatricians, community children's nurses, social workers, housing officers, support groups and charities and, of course, GPs.

Once diagnosis is established and the scope of the challenge identified we also take on a liaison and educational role. We make contact with schools and kids' groups like Brownies and football clubs to ensure that members of staff understand how to keep your child safe and are trained in emergency treatment.

So all in all, your health visitor can be a very useful supporter and source of advice for you and your family through an often difficult and challenging time. It is up to you to make contact with your health visitor and share your concerns. We can be contacted through the local surgery or medical centre and are always happy to help in any way we can.

In the beginning we were very stressed at times, either because we were not getting the help we needed or because we were overwhelmed by what was happening and the effect it had on our lives. Most people prepare for a child to change their lives but we could not have prepared ourselves for this. Dawn

Paediatricians

Your GP may initially refer your child to a paediatrician at your nearest hospital for assessment. This is often the case in areas where there is no specialist allergy clinic. The paediatrician, who is a specialist in childhood illnesses, will be able to give an overview of all the problems connected with your child's allergies. In many cases the paediatrician will be able to treat your child themselves. Alternatively, he or she may decide to refer you to an allergy specialist.

The paediatrician should already have the relevant notes from your GP but will still want to hear the full history of your child's allergies. Once again, write your questions down to take to the appointment, and do not be afraid to ask anything, no matter how irrelevant it may seem.

If your GP has not suggested that you be referred to a paediatrician you can always ask if this would be useful.

Paediatrician Dr Andrew Boon describes his role in diagnosing and treating allergy:

The main role of the paediatrician is to listen carefully to the parents' description of the child's symptoms. It is sometimes quite difficult to determine whether symptoms, particularly a rash, are due to an allergic reaction or to some other cause. Most district general hospitals do not have a full time paediatric allergy service and there will be limited facilities for allergy testing. Nevertheless, many paediatricians will be able to offer limited allergy testing. For some allergies such as cow's milk in babies, allergy testing is not particularly helpful and the paediatrician may advise dietary restrictions such as cutting out cow's milk on the basis of the history alone. All paediatric departments should have a paediatric dietitian who will be able to give advice about any special diet.

The paediatrician should be able to manage most allergies but if the child has complex, severe or life-threatening allergies (anaphylaxis), a referral will usually be made to a specialist allergy clinic for further investigations and advice about the management of the allergy.

At the hospital they talked about allergens but I must admit I didn't really understand. They said they could do testing and that we might have to carry around an injector pen if it was that severe. They told me all this but there was no referral or anything. I really wanted someone to tell me, 'If this has happened to you, these are the steps you need to take next' and I wanted to understand why people react to certain foods. Alison

Allergy specialists

If you are fortunate, you may be referred to one of the few allergy clinics where your child can be seen for all their tests, eczema, asthma and dietary advice at one visit. The majority of parents, however, will have to take an allergic child to a different clinic for each problem and travel considerable distances. Inevitably this is difficult and time consuming. Finding ways to control your own stress in order to make the most of each appointment is important.

- Write down the questions you want to ask.
- Take a pad and pen to write down the answers.
- Take somebody else with you. If your partner cannot attend, see if a family member or a close friend will come along. Two pairs of ears are better than one.
- An extra pair of hands also leaves you free to concentrate fully on what the specialist is saying while someone else looks after your child or children.

Allergy clinics are spread thinly and unevenly round the country. There are a small number of major centres staffed by full-time allergy specialists, a few part-time centres and many more part-time allergy clinics run by consultants in other medical specialities. NHS waiting lists can be months long, depending on your area. This situation is not ideal but is being addressed by the NHS and allergy support groups.

In order to see an allergy specialist quickly you may choose to pay for a private consultation. Be aware that you will be charged for the consultation, tests and any medications prescribed. You can ask the receptionist in advance what these will cost. If you have existing private health insurance some, if not all, of these costs may be covered. Also be aware that private appointments at an NHS hospital may be outside normal hours if the specialist is fitting these in around the NHS clinics.

Specialists are extremely busy, seeing as many patients as possible during each clinic. They will be pleased to see somebody who has come prepared and is clear about what they want to know. (See also *Allergy testing* p.44.) If the specialist seems remote or unapproachable, do not be put off. Stick to your questions and ask him or her to explain again anything that you don't immediately understand.

On the whole our experience of health professionals has been good, although we had to be insistent and determined early on in order to get the right people to listen. Our GP was knowledgeable, already having a very allergic child on her books. She was able to refer us quickly to Southampton Hospital under Professor Warner. He proved to be extremely helpful in treating Lorie's eczema and identifying and coping with her multiple allergies. Tom

Allergy specialist Dr Richard Turner describes his role:

My approach is holistic as allergy can affect many different parts of the body and symptoms can be diverse. Therefore it is important to give enough time (often an hour) for a consultation. This, coupled with too few paediatric allergy specialists, means waiting times for appointments are longer than I, and many of my fellow specialists, would like.

I send every parent a questionnaire to complete prior to the appointment ensuring they have time to be accurate about the answers. It also gives them time to ask relatives about unknown family history and get details from separated spouses, for example.

At the appointment, I go through the details of the child's medical history and clarify the exact details of the symptoms described. Then an allergy nurse does the appropriate skin-prick testing. The skin-prick tests take 15 minutes to react. A positive reaction will take a maximum of two hours to disappear.

Immediately after these tests the patient returns to see me. I then try to interpret the history and testing into definite, probable or no proven allergy. If I can only diagnose a probable allergy I may need to ask the parent to do more detective work at which stage a blood test may be included. Sometimes, if it is still unclear whether a certain food is causing a problem, then a food challenge is done by trying small quantities of the food thought to be causing the problem to see if in reality it does, in the safety of a day case unit (at the hospital). This is the best way to test the absence of a food allergy but often needs a two hour appointment.

If an allergy is diagnosed, I discuss various ways of managing it under three headings: appropriate avoidance of allergens; appropriate use of local treatments; appropriate use of oral drugs.

Hopefully, at the end of the consultation, using the treatments suggested the problems the patient came with will be lessened, making his or her life more comfortable.

At the beginning I wanted to know things that people couldn't tell me – like when Matthew was going to grow out of it. You just want to be given a little bit of light at the end of the tunnel. Gwyneth

Dietitians

A dietitian will help you to devise a diet for your child that is both safe and nutritionally balanced. You may be asked to keep a food diary for one or two weeks (p.77) enabling the dietitian to analyse your child's intake and advise you on changes so that your child receives the right nutrients. If your child has to avoid a number of foods, supplements will be suggested to ensure a healthy, balanced diet. For example, children who are allergic to dairy products need to have their calcium intake assessed because even if you use calcium enriched soya milk, a calcium supplement is likely to be needed.

One of the things that worried me most in the early days was whether he was getting enough calcium, vitamins and iron etc. for healthy growth. Dawn

You are entitled to see a dietitian so don't forget to ask if your doctor fails to suggest it. If you are getting it right, the dietitian will give you welcome reassurance. If you are struggling, the dietitian will give you valuable guidance on evolving a balanced diet to accommodate your child's particular allergies. He or she may also be able to suggest alternative foods and recipes that you have not even considered. He or she can also discuss issues such as how to deal with 'may contain' labelling and how to keep your child safe in different situations.

The hospital dietitian turned out to be the most splendid friend in those early months. Dawn

I found the dietitian we saw at the hospital unhelpful. She knew very little about allergy. To see someone else I would have had to ring up Zac's specialist and tell her that I wasn't happy with the dietitian she had referred me to. It all felt too uncomfortable and I wasn't sure she would be able to refer me to someone else anyway – all very awkward. Looking back, I wish I had. I now know that there are excellent allergy dietitians out there. Alice

If you are not receiving adequate advice or need more than that dietitian can offer, look for one who specialises in allergy, with the help of your child's specialist or GP. You can expect to return to the dietitian for reviews. How often you visit is up to you and the dietitian.

TOP TIP Making a list of the foods your family likes to eat will help the dietician devise a diet to suit your shopping and cooking habits.

Dietitian Debbie Evans describes her role in children's food allergy:

- To ensure that the child's diet is nutritionally adequate for all nutrients as far as possible.
- To advise on avoiding allergens. This includes detecting allergens on food labels and food products.
- To advise on making the restricted diet as palatable as possible, for example, advice on the most appropriate milk substitutes if milk is to be avoided or bread substitutes if wheat is avoided.
- To give advice on specialist food and drink items available in supermarkets, health food shops, through specialist companies and on prescription.
- To give advice on following the restricted diet on a day-to-day basis and in special circumstances such as holidays.
- To liaise with other health professionals and agencies (such as schools) as appropriate to help make sure the family is supported appropriately.

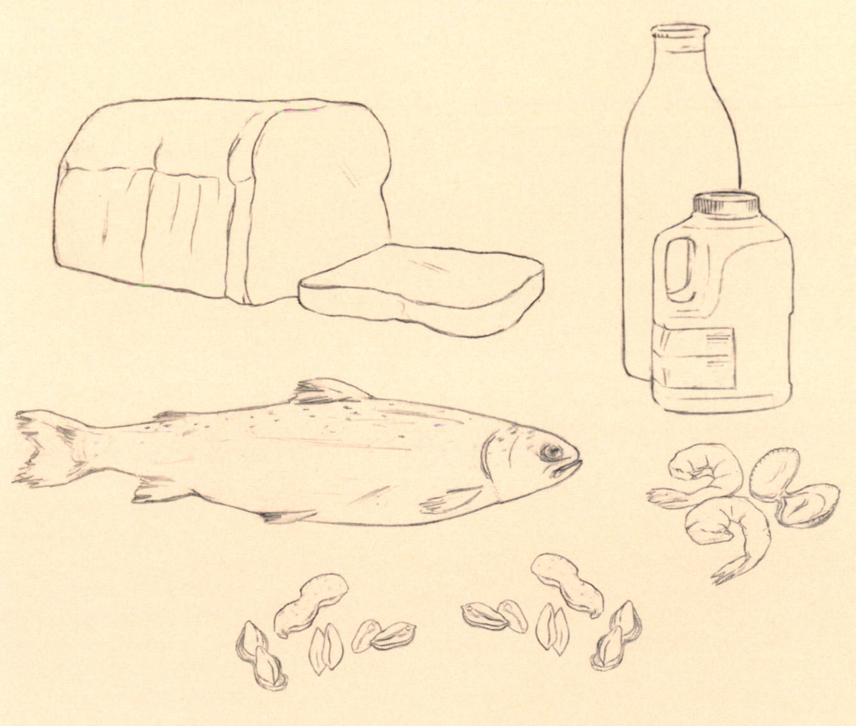

2 Food allergy or food intolerance?

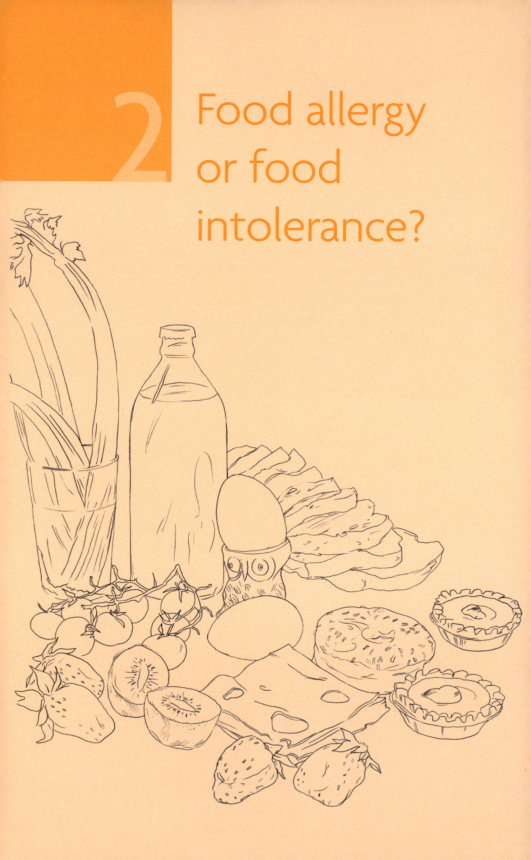

Food allergy is a disease that involves the immune system and which can, in its most severe form, lead to the sudden death of an otherwise healthy person.

Food intolerance is the term used to cover reactions where the immune system has no proven role in the symptoms and is more common than food allergy. Although symptoms can be severe and very distressing they are not potentially fatal.

Professor John O. Warner highlights an important difference, 'Food allergy will occur with only tiny doses of the offending food whereas, in general, food intolerance only occurs with moderate to large doses. For instance, those babies who have lactose intolerance will only react when they have moderate to large quantities, whereas if they are milk allergic they can react to minute amounts. While food intolerance in general does not cause life-threatening reactions, it can sometimes be very severe and seriously compromise health, leading to chronic, severe problems. This is very obvious in relation to coeliac disease. Thus, while it may not be life-threatening in the short term, theoretically it could be in the long term.'

In mainstream medicine there is a clear distinction between allergy and intolerance and it will be easier to communicate with your doctor if you too understand these definitions. It is not unknown for a parent to talk in terms of their child's allergies when in fact the problem is food intolerance. In cases where a doctor is not especially sympathetic, this kind of confusion can lead to fraught exchanges and a breakdown in communication with the very person from whom you need help most.

Is this food intolerance?

The symptoms of food intolerance in children can be awful and debilitating in their own right and can include nausea; bloating; abdominal pain or discomfort; diarrhoea; constipation; respiratory problems; rashes; glue ear; palpitations; headaches; joint pains; sweating; and cystitis. Symptoms can vary daily, and can occur hours if not days after eating the food which makes finding out which food is responsible difficult.

Allergy tests such as skin-prick and RAST (p.44) can only help your doctor to diagnose intolerance by *ruling out* allergy. Working out by trial and error which foods your child can and cannot tolerate will be a long process. But careful management of food intolerance can make a huge difference to a child's quality of life so it is worth persevering.

We recommend reading *The Complete Guide to Food Allergy and Intolerance* (Appendix). This is an excellent, in-depth look at intolerance accompanied by case histories and guidance on elimination diets for children. It also contains a detailed breakdown of food groups.

One of the most common complaints from sufferers of food intolerance is that people are sceptical about the problem, even suggesting that it is all in the mind (psychosomatic). Comments of this sort are even more annoying when it is your child who is suffering. You know they're not 'faking it', but you may be made to feel like a neurotic parent and even start to doubt your own judgement. Our advice is to remain calm, keep a food and symptoms diary (p.77) and persevere with your doctor. We suggest that you use the word 'intolerance' or 'sensitivity', rather than 'allergy', to describe your child's symptoms until an accurate diagnosis has been made.

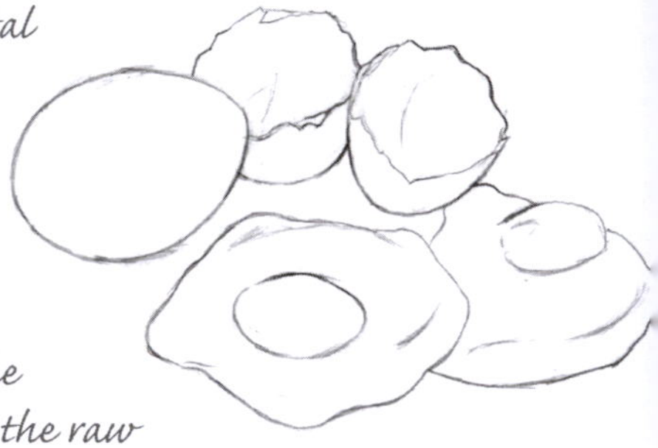

We enrolled in a food study at a local hospital which was being undertaken to establish why some people grow out of egg allergies and why some don't. We spent a day in the research centre at the hospital where Katie was treated like royalty. As we knew that she could already tolerate baked egg the consultant was happy to progress straight to the raw egg challenge.

Katie behaved beautifully throughout and was a very co-operative and amenable patient. About 5 hours after we arrived, we were told that as she had not reacted to any part of the testing, she no longer had an egg allergy. What a relief! However, despite seeing all the testing in front of my own eyes I was still in a state of disbelief and denial. Did that really mean she could eat egg now? The doctor's advice was to give her small quantities of egg initially and increase the quantities slowly to build our confidence.

So I came home from hospital elated and on a real high. However it was short lived as she was sick several times on the night of the testing, and was pretty poorly with sickness and diarrhoea for the next 4 days. I spoke to the study team who thought that although the tests proved she no longer had a life threatening allergy to egg, the sickness and diarrhoea looked likely to indicate that she has an intolerance to egg. The only way to be sure would be feed her reasonable quantities of egg a couple more times to see if each occasion resulted in more sickness and diarrhoea. To date that has been rather tricky, as Katie seems to have an in-built aversion to all egg products and no amount of coercing and cajoling seems to be able to bribe her into even trying the smallest amount of boiled, scrambled, fried or any other type of egg.

I do feel glad to have been part of the study and I won't need to worry about the contents of school dinners or need to watch what she eats at birthday parties or worry about entrusting the medication to mothers of school friends who might invite her home for tea. And at the end of the day there are lots of people who choose not to eat certain foods because it makes them unwell, which is certainly a lot easier to live with than a potentially fatal allergy. Tracy

Is this an allergic reaction or a common childhood illness?

Not every rash your child develops will be due to allergy, nor will every tummy ache, bout of diarrhoea or vomiting. There are many childhood illnesses which share these symptoms, from the simplest heat-rash through to more serious conditions. For parents who are used to looking out for allergic reactions it is easy to fall into the trap of assuming that symptoms are allergic.

Sarah had been eating some very colourful sweets prior to developing an itchy rash across her body. I gave her antihistamine, read to see what colourings in the sweets could have caused the rash and lectured Sarah about colourings and additives. The rash lasted a week and when I finally took her to the doctor, it turned out that she had a virus and was then off school unwell for three weeks. That's when I realised I really had to remember not to put everything down to allergy. Deborah

A number of common childhood illnesses share many of the same symptoms as an allergic reaction. If you are in any doubt, the information below may help you decide.

- Severe allergic reactions will usually occur within minutes of the offending food being eaten and escalate quickly. The symptoms are usually so clear that it is obvious what is happening. It is hard to confuse anaphylaxis with anything else (pp.33 & 38).
- With milder symptoms, however, it may be more difficult to differentiate between allergy and illness because the reaction may be less immediate, developing up to two hours later.
- If, before going to the doctor, you are trying to determine whether symptoms are due to allergy or illness, take your child's temperature. If he or she is ill his or her body temperature may well be rising whereas an allergic reaction is not normally accompanied by a rise in temperature (although your child may look sweaty with an allergic reaction).
- Remember too that allergic symptoms should improve with a dose of antihistamine, such as Piriton. It's worth pointing out that the correct dose of antihistamine given when it is not actually needed will not harm your child.
- If at any time you do become anxious about the symptoms or are in doubt about how to treat your child, telephone your doctor's surgery or NHS Direct for advice.

3 Medical terminology explained

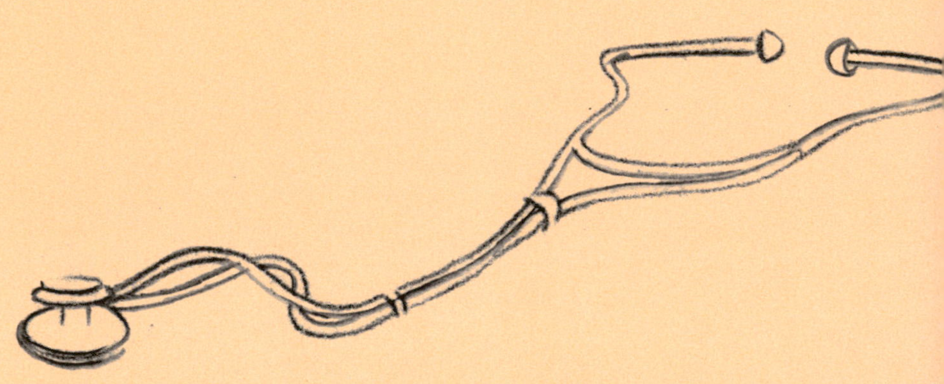

In this section we explain the medical terminology your doctor may use to describe symptoms associated with allergies. (A glossary is also provided on p.14.)

Atopic

Being atopic means that you are likely to suffer from allergies because of your genetic make-up. Allergies themselves are not passed from generation to generation but the genetic predisposition (being likely to have an allergy) is. If you are atopic it does not necessarily mean you will develop allergies, which is why some children from allergic families never develop allergies.

We have some family history of allergies. Lorie's aunt has multiple allergies, including latex, anaesthetics and bananas. I have hay fever but my wife, Lilly, has no allergies. Tom

We both have hay fever and as a child I was allergic to milk and am still intolerant to meat, fish and egg. My husband, Barry, had dreadful eczema and asthma as a child, being hospitalised several times. Dawn

We are quite an allergic family but have no history of food allergy, other than my son having a mild reaction (urticaria) to strawberries when he was about four but never before or since. I have had asthma and hay fever since I was tiny and my son has hay fever and eczema. Katie's had mild eczema since she was a baby. Tracy

Gastrointestinal symptoms

These are symptoms of the stomach and gut. They can begin as soon as the offending food is put into the mouth or up to several hours later.

- **Stomach cramps (colic)** means pain in the abdomen caused by muscle spasm and trapped wind, and may be mild or extreme.
- **Nausea** (feeling sick) and **vomiting** (being sick). Your child may just feel sick but violent vomiting is a common first reaction to ingesting an allergen and can be very distressing.
- **Diarrhoea** can be an immediate reaction to an allergen accompanied by vomiting, or may take a little longer to develop and can be accompanied by painful stomach cramps.
- **Oral Allergy Syndrome** sufferers describe tingling, itching and soreness in the mouth on eating certain fruits and vegetables. It can be linked to hay fever and often occurs seasonally. Fruit and vegetable proteins are altered by heat and Oral Allergy Syndrome sufferers sometimes find that they can tolerate them cooked but not raw.

Cutaneous reactions

Cutaneous means 'of the skin', so these are reactions which affect internal and external skin tissue.

- **Urticaria** is also known as hives or nettle rash because it resembles nettle stings: itchy lumps which are white with red surrounding tissue. It can occur anywhere on the body but most commonly around the mouth and on the face and hands. It may continue to appear elsewhere on the body as the allergen is digested.
- **Angioedema.** Swellings, most commonly on the lips, eyelids and tongue, which can be large – often painful rather than itchy.
- **Tingling and itching of the lips and tongue** are often the first indication that something is wrong. A very young child might rub furiously at his or her lips.
- **Eczema** is a skin condition characterised by redness and small blisters. It may take as long as 72 hours to appear and last for some time.
- **Pruritus** means any intense sensation of itching.

Respiratory symptoms

These are symptoms that affect the airways.

- **Stridor** is the particular noise of breathing due to inflammation of the larynx (throat). It can sound like hoarseness.
- **Choking cough.** A child may begin to cough as if some food has become 'stuck' due to inflammation of the larynx (throat).
- **Wheezing.** As the airways are irritated they become narrowed making it harder to breathe. This causes the characteristic 'wheezy' sound of asthma.
- **Laboured breathing.** If further swelling of the mouth and airways occurs and continues, it will become increasingly difficult to breathe. The child may try to breathe in gasps and gulps, swallowing air as quickly as possible.
- **Cyanosis.** The child may begin to look blue, especially around the lips because there is not enough oxygen in the blood.

Coughing, wheezing and laboured breathing can all be symptoms of an asthma attack even if no food has been eaten. If you suspect that your child may be having an asthma attack, seek medical help immediately.

Circulatory symptoms

These are symptoms affecting the blood, blood pressure and circulation.

- **Sweating.** An allergic reaction can cause the child to feel uncomfortably hot and he or she may sweat more than usual. By contrast, the child might feel cold and clammy to the touch.
- **Hypotension** means abnormally low blood pressure.

- **Collapse** is due to a drop in blood pressure. During a severe allergic reaction the total volume of blood circulating around the body is drastically reduced because the blood vessels in the tissues dilate and become leaky, so less blood returns to the heart to be pumped round the body. This causes blood pressure to drop, making it difficult for the heart to pump enough blood to all the vital organs. The result will be dizziness, fainting, eye-rolling and even loss of consciousness.

Anaphylaxis

Anaphylaxis is the term used to describe a severe allergic reaction affecting the whole body that in its most extreme form (anaphylactic shock) can be fatal.

An anaphylactic reaction is the result of a powerful cocktail of chemicals, including histamine, being released into the body from cells in the blood and the tissues, called mast cells. Mast cells are primed to respond to invasion by substances that may be harmful to the body. In the case of allergy they mistakenly react to a harmless substance, such as food, with inappropriate force.

People who have suffered anaphylactic reactions describe some or all of the following symptoms:

An anaphylactic reaction is alarming to see, mostly because of the speed with which it occurs. It is impossible to say quite how your child will react as the progression of symptoms is different for everyone.

Flushing of the skin Hives (nettle rash) and itching, especially of the face and hands Angioedema – swelling of the lips, mouth, face, tongue, throat, hands and feet	Due to leakiness and relaxation of the small blood vessels
Stomach cramps Vomiting or diarrhoea	Due to muscle spasms in the gut
Hoarseness Difficulty in swallowing or speaking Difficulty breathing, wheezing	Due to muscle spasms and narrowing of the airways in the lungs
Alterations in heart rate (palpitations) Sudden feeling of weakness, faintness Anxiety or sense of impending doom Collapse and unconsciousness	Due to leakiness and relaxation of the larger blood vessels that supply and collect blood from the heart and other major organs, resulting in falling blood pressure

We were on holiday in Cornwall in a remote village. It was Boxing Day 1997 and Lorie was six months old. For breakfast that morning we fed her a little (pea-sized) scrambled egg. Within five to ten minutes she started crying. Thinking she was tired, we laid her in her cot. Within minutes she was violently sick, her face and hands swelled up in a red rash and her body went limp. Her breathing was also laboured (we now know she was experiencing anaphylactic shock). We called the emergency services, but it was quicker for us to travel in our car to the surgery some 20 minutes away. The doctor was very good and immediately realised it was a very severe allergic reaction to food. We knew that egg was the only new food Lorie had eaten that morning. It was an extremely worrying and anxious time. We did panic at one stage and thought we might lose her when she started breathing erratically, going limp and turning blue. We felt really helpless. Lilly

I was feeding Fay. Jake went into the kitchen and helped himself to my biscuit, which I had left at the back of the worktop, out of reach I thought. Jake took one bite, just one small bite, and said, 'Hmm, yum biscuit.' A second later he began to cough. I quickly got up to check on him and saw the biscuit in his hand. He was already becoming distressed. I gave him 3mls of Piriton (antihistamine) which he vomited up almost immediately. I knew I had to get him to hospital as at this time I didn't have adrenaline injectors for him, so I picked up the baby and changing bag and put them in the car. Then I put Jake in too. All the time he was becoming more agitated, his skin was covered in urticaria and his face, mouth and tongue were swelling. He was beginning to wheeze and finding it difficult to talk. I kept talking to him, pressing him to answer me. He did his best but lost consciousness. It must have taken about ten minutes for him to fall unconscious and just a little longer to get him to casualty at the hospital. They put him onto oxygen immediately and gave him a large dose of Piriton. He stayed in hospital until 7pm and it took him another two days to feel well enough to eat; it was the following day before he wanted to play. Dawn

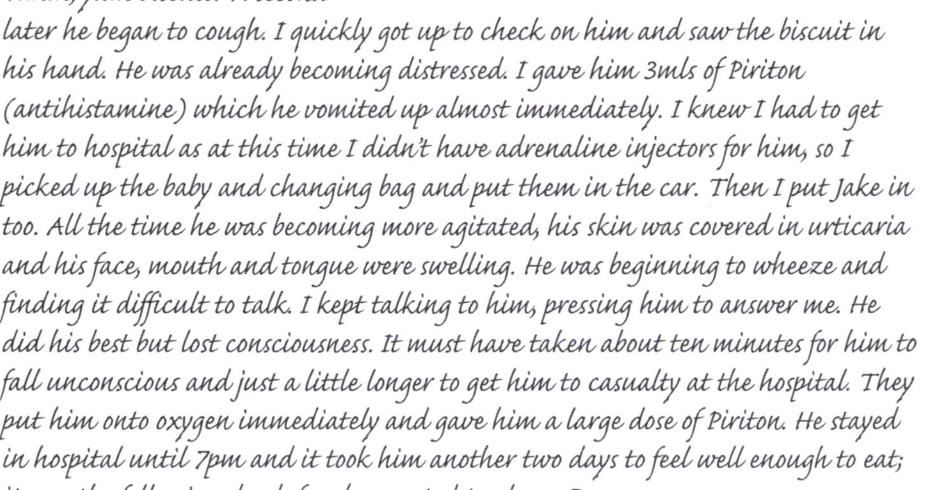

When Peter had an anaphylactic reaction he came up in hives, followed by extreme tiredness and wheezing, falling asleep and needing antihistamine and oxygen to revive him. This only happened once and it was at hospital under controlled conditions. Peter was given 10mls of Piriton and then an oxygen mask for half an hour. He was then monitored for another two hours. Angela

Sometimes we noticed that Alex's face would become blotchy and red after eating. One lunch time his nursery rang to say he had had some sort of allergic reaction, that his face was covered in a red rash and that he was very unsettled. We worked out over a fairly long period of time that the blotchiness was linked with peas and green beans, so we simply avoided them. This was fine until November last year. I stupidly let Alex dip some bread in my fresh vegetable soup. He put the bread to his mouth and then spat it back into my bowl (much to my annoyance).

The speed of the reaction was frightening. He came out in blisters all around his lips and mouth, his face went very red, and his breathing was affected. He started to cry, saying his tummy hurt and went from being perfectly fine to looking really unwell. I panicked and really didn't know what to do. Should I use Daisy's adrenaline auto-injector or assume the reaction would calm down? In the end I decided I couldn't risk it and phoned for an ambulance. They came very fast and decided to take him in to hospital.

The reaction had started to calm down a bit, but they were concerned that his mouth and throat were covered in tiny blisters. Alex loves ambulances but was feeling so poorly that he hardly took any notice. By the time we reached the hospital he was a lot calmer and almost back to his normal self (he started going on and on about the ambulance!). They checked him over and decided to keep us in for an hour to make sure he didn't have a further reaction. Then we were sent home with a bottle of antihistamine. Alison

Which foods can cause anaphylaxis?

Any food, is the rather alarming answer. In *children* the most common allergens are cow's milk, eggs, peanuts, tree nuts (almonds, hazelnuts, walnuts, cashews, pecans, Brazils, pistachios, macadamia nuts and Queensland nuts), fish, shellfish, soya and wheat which make up 98% of all childhood allergens. The other 2% is made up of rarer allergens.

4 Adrenaline auto-injectors

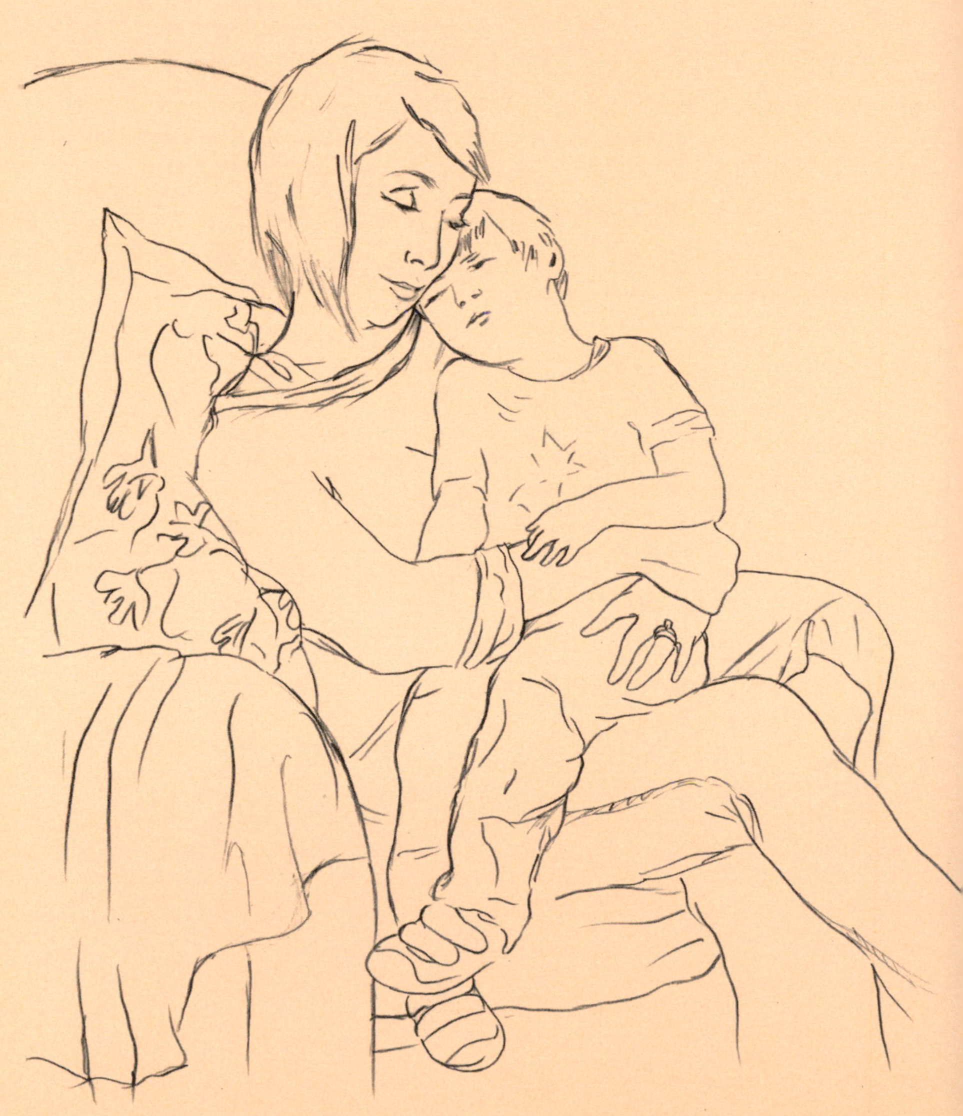

Adrenaline (epinephrine)

Adrenaline is a life-saver for those with anaphylaxis because it works instantly to reverse the symptoms of an anaphylactic reaction.

During anaphylaxis, blood vessels leak, bronchial tissues swell and blood pressure drops, causing choking and collapse. Adrenaline (epinephrine) acts quickly to constrict blood vessels, relax smooth muscles in the lungs to improve breathing, stimulate the heartbeat and help to stop swelling around the face and lips.   Anaphylaxis Campaign

If your child has already had an anaphylactic reaction or is considered at risk of anaphylaxis, he or she will have been prescribed adrenaline auto-injectors, which make it easy to inject adrenaline in an emergency. The doctor should show you how to use the device they prescribe. In the UK, Anapen and EpiPen are the trade names for spring-activated auto-injectors containing a sterile single dose of adrenaline. They both do the same job although the design and the way you use them differs slightly. Both brands are available on NHS prescription. If you'd like more detail on the differences please look at their websites.

Dosage

Anapens and EpiPens are available in two different strengths:

Adult: delivers 0.3mg of adrenaline and is suitable for those over 30kg (4st 10lb)
Junior: delivers 0.15mg of adrenaline and is suitable for children 15-30kg (2st 5lb – 4st 10lb)

Since children reach 30kg at varying ages, weight determines when it is time to move on to the adult adrenaline auto-injector. Weigh your child regularly if he or she is approaching 30kg so that you can be sure the dosage is appropriate. Double-check that you have been prescribed the correct dosage for your child.

Babies under 15kg

When babies who weigh less than 15kg are diagnosed with anaphylaxis, you may be prescribed phials of adrenaline that you can draw up yourself with a syringe. This sounds worrying but you can be taught by the nurse how to administer adrenaline safely this way. Practise on an orange with a spare syringe, using water instead of adrenaline, to get used to the technique. Remember to dispose of used syringes responsibly and to use a new, sterile syringe each time, as indicated by your nurse.

TOP TIP

It is better to give an unnecessary dose of adrenaline than not to have used it when it was needed. Always carry adrenaline auto-injectors and know how to use them.

Using an adrenaline auto-injector

Anapens and EpiPens make the administration of the life-saving medicine your child needs as easy as it possibly could be.

In *theory* it is simple to give the right dose of adrenaline by following the standard instructions on the device. However, in *practice* it doesn't always feel that easy!

Max (7) came out of the play area saying that he didn't feel very well and that he was really hot. I took him out into the fresh air but, by the time we had got outside he couldn't see very well or walk any more. I had him cuddled up on my lap and was asking him if his stomach hurt or if anywhere on his body did and he pointed to his throat. I started to notice that he was getting hotter and that his skin was changing colour.

I said to my sister that I thought he was having an anaphylactic shock and we might need help, so she went to a member of staff who called for first aid. By the time she got back Max had started to drift away and was like a rag doll on me and it was difficult to keep hold of him. I was really starting to panic and trying to make myself keep calm. I told my sister I thought he might need his adrenaline pen and she got one out. A crowd of adults and children had started to gather around us.

The first-aiders arrived very quickly and my sister told them what the problem was. Max had got worse by this time and was hardly responding to me. That's when my sister said that I should give him the adrenaline injection but all these people were looking at him and he was suffering so badly, I just wanted to hug him and hide him from everyone. Then the first-aider also said that I should do it, but I just couldn't put him through any more stress. I was thinking, 'What if it doesn't work and he goes through more pain for nothing?' Then my sister volunteered to do it and I showed her where to inject him whilst I was still hugging him.

When she put the injection into him he screamed and my sister started to count to ten quite loudly. By the time she got to five Max started to hug me back as he started coming back to me.

This all happened within five minutes.

Now I know how quickly and brilliantly the adrenaline works, I hope that if there is a next time I will use it much more quickly. Amanda

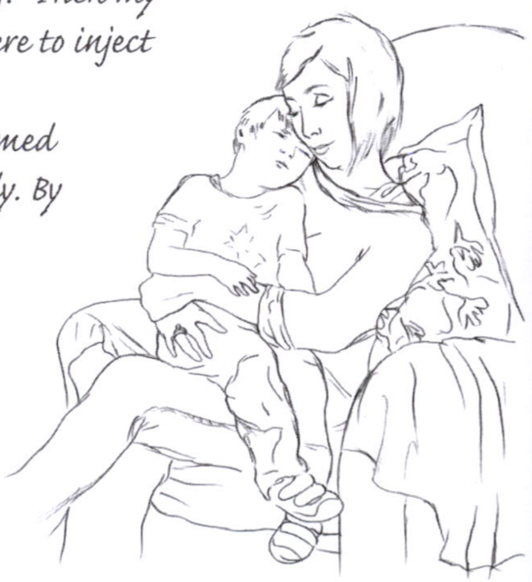

Thomas was 15 months old when he had his first anaphylactic shock. He had reached up onto the counter and taken a sip of his sister's milk.

He went really white and his lips turned blue. Hives were appearing all over his body and then his eyes starting rolling up. This was all happening right there in front of me and then he went all floppy. It was all happening so fast. I stood there for what felt like ages knowing I had to find the adrenaline. I think I hesitated because there was no swelling which I'd expected. Then my brain clicked into gear and I realised he must be having a huge drop in blood pressure and collapsing. I picked him up, ran to find his adrenaline pens and had to get one out of its box with Thomas in my arms. I ended up using my teeth to pull the lid off the tube and take off the safety cap because I had this floppy toddler in my arms and an EpiPen in my hand not knowing how to co-ordinate it all.

I sat down on the sofa so I could use my body to support him, yanked his trousers down with my left hand and put the injector against his thigh with my right. I paused to be sure I really needed to do this before pressing but I knew I had to. As soon as I did he screamed out and jerked his body in reaction which I wasn't really expecting – I had to hold him really tight while he writhed, still holding the injector pen against him, and count to ten.

When I pulled the adrenaline pen away I was really shocked to see the needle. I'm not sure why because I obviously knew there would be one, I just hadn't thought in advance about the fact that I'd be pulling it out of his leg! So there I was now with a wriggly crying toddler in one arm and a needle in the other. I must have put it down. I was shaking badly and thinking I just don't know what to do but in my head I knew I had to phone an ambulance next. Thomas was then sick all over the floor but he was getting his colour back and I knew he would be okay. The adrenaline had saved his life. Once the ambulance was on its way I just collapsed into an armchair with him and had a good cry.

The first time is definitely the worst. Even though you prepare yourself for anaphylactic shock, it's still so scary and unexpected when it happens. Having practised a few times with a trainer pen really helped me when I had to do it for real. Deborah

You are likely to be shaky after administering the injection and your child needs to be cuddled and reassured after such a frightening experience. In fact, you'll both need a big hug.

Always dial 999 after using the adrenaline auto-injector

In most cases the adrenaline will work immediately and recovery will be swift. It is still important however to dial 999 rather than drive your child to hospital yourself. Not only do paramedics carry the necessary equipment to deal with further deterioration or a relapse, they can also get you to the hospital fast and straight into casualty.

How many adrenaline auto-injectors does my child need?

At least **two**. Allergy specialists advise carrying two adrenaline auto-injectors in case a second injection is required before the patient reaches hospital or one is damaged. The most important thing to remember is that wherever your child is there must be at least two injectors close by in case they have a reaction. Good nurseries, schools and doctors are clued up and will insist on having two adrenaline auto-injectors on site permanently.

Q: *My daughter starts school next term and the head teacher has asked us to provide two adrenaline auto-injectors to keep on site. Do I ask my doctor for two more or should I take my daughter's adrenaline auto-injectors in every day?*

A: Doctors usually prescribe extra adrenaline auto-injectors when a child starts school. They appreciate that the school needs to be sure that your child's medication is readily available. If you have any problems, the school may be willing to write a letter explaining their requirement for medication to be held on site.

Q: *My child spends four days a week at her grandparents. I would like to keep two adrenaline auto-injectors at their house but my doctor refuses to prescribe extras because they are so expensive. He says that we must take the two we already have back and forth. Is there anything I can do?*

A: Adrenaline auto-injectors are considered expensive partly because they are a 'just in case' medication and because the expiry dates can come round quickly. This does eat into a GP's stretched budget. Many doctors argue that so few children will ever actually need their adrenaline auto-injectors that unless there are special circumstances, your doctor is likely to consider that two is sufficient. You could offer to pay for the extra adrenaline auto-injectors yourself. However, it is worth remembering that learning to carry adrenaline auto-injectors with your child at all times is a necessary part of living with anaphylaxis. It can be safer than keeping the medication in different places because you may forget to carry yours with you on the journey to her grandparents or when just popping out, for example. This is an on-going problem for families with anaphylactic children.

Q: *We've never had to use our adrenaline auto-injectors and I worry that I won't know when to use it or that I might give it when she doesn't really need it. How will I know?*

A: This is a common concern among parents. In fact, it is very unlikely that you'll be in any doubt as severe symptoms are hard to mistake for anything else. The advice from doctors is that it is better to give an unnecessary dose of adrenaline than not to have used it when it was needed. The paramedics can also give you guidance on the spot. Just stay calm, and keep monitoring your child.

Trainer pens

Trainer pens contain no needle or adrenaline but in all other regards function just like the real thing. They are *extremely* useful for you and anybody else who looks after your child to practise with. Both Anapen and EpiPen make trainer pens (Appendix). Ask your doctor, health visitor or school's nurse to order one for you.

Teaching other people to use adrenaline auto-injectors

Allow plenty of time to show someone else how to use the adrenaline auto-injector and to answer any questions. Most people will never have seen or handled one before. You may like to buy a trainer pen (see above) so other people can get used to how it works. Here's a checklist to go through with them:

1. **Show them** how to operate the pen, pointing out the instructions on the side of the pen for reference.
2. **Show them** where to administer the injection – into the thickest part of the thigh (through clothing is fine).
3. **Tell them** how to identify an allergic reaction, what symptoms to look out for in your child and when it is appropriate to use the adrenaline auto-injector.
4. **Back all this up** with brief, written instructions on what to do in an emergency and your contact telephone numbers.

TOP TIP

Learn how to use your chosen adrenaline auto-injector. Teach other people effectively. Reminding people that they need to follow the clear instructions on the adrenaline auto-injector is a good habit to form.

Talk about idiotic! Once, when I was in a bit of a hurry showing a friend how to use Sophie's adrenaline, I grabbed what I thought was the trainer pen and ended up injecting myself in the leg with the real thing. I screamed out in shock and surprise then fell about giggling and felt completely hyper and light headed for the rest of the day – well you would after a shot of adrenaline! So much for the competent mother! I haven't lived that one down yet. Jackie

Trainer pens are a great way to familiarise yourself, and anyone else, with your child's adrenaline auto-injectors. Professor John O. Warner says, 'If there is any doubt about whether adrenaline should be used, then it should be used. Problems are infinitely more likely to occur as a consequence of failure to use adrenaline if an anaphylactic reaction is developing. Clearly however it is important to follow the guidelines on its use as issued by the prescriber. An unnecessary dose is highly unlikely to do any harm in a healthy individual.'

Common reactions from other people:

Q: *Will I hurt your child?*

A: No. If the adrenaline auto-injector is needed then the child will already be in a state of distress or losing consciousness. Not only will the child barely notice the injection but you will be saving his or her life.

Q: *I'm frightened of needles and injections, will I be able to do it?*

A: Don't worry – this isn't like most other injections. This is a pre-loaded device, with the needle concealed inside the pen so you won't see it. However, after using the adrenaline auto-injector, there will be a short needle sticking out at the end of the device. Put the used adrenaline auto-injector back in its case, needle first, and give it to the paramedic.

Q: *What if I lose my nerve or do it wrong?*

A: Ask what is worrying them and discuss any fears. You have to accept that some people will feel unable to take on the responsibility. Better that you find out now.

Q: *How will I remember to do things in the right order?*

A: Remind them that you have written it all down in numbered steps with a clear description of signs of anaphylaxis in your child. Explain that they will not be alone – either they will have you on the other end of the phone or they will have called 999 and the ambulance crew will talk them through what needs to be done.

There is a fine line between scaring somebody and giving them adequate information to recognise and treat an anaphylactic reaction. For anyone other than the parents, it requires a fair degree of courage to accept that there may be a situation where he or she may need to give an injection. It may help to remind a carer that by using the adrenaline auto-injector, what they are actually doing is *saving a life*.

Protecting adrenaline auto-injectors

I find the bum bags and tough tubes sold to carry and protect adrenaline auto-injectors really useful, especially when Zac hurls his satchel around the school playground. Alice

Bum bags and tough plastic tubes to carry and protect adrenaline auto-injectors are available from YellowCross, Medicare Plus and Kidsaware (Appendix).

To prevent the adrenaline deteriorating, auto-injectors should always be stored at room temperature and away from the light. They should not be exposed to dramatic temperature changes and should never be stored near a source of heat, in the fridge or allowed to freeze. If this happens accidentally, replace them.

Expiry dates and reminders

Anapen and EpiPen both run Expiry Date Alert services. Fill out the forms enclosed with the devices. They will automatically send you a reminder a month before expiry.

Golden rules:

Check that:

- Wherever your child goes two adrenaline auto-injectors go too.
- You know how to use the adrenaline auto-injectors – practise with trainer pens.
- Other carers know how to recognise an allergic reaction and administer adrenaline.
- Any asthma medication is carried on the child at all times.
- Medication is in date and not damaged.
- You replace the adrenaline auto-injectors at the earliest possible opportunity when they've been used.
- You carry a mobile phone, fully charged and with plenty of credit.

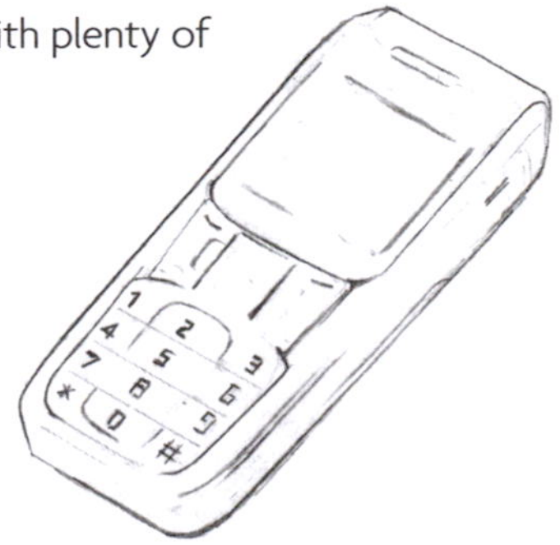

IN THE BEGINNING

5 Allergy testing

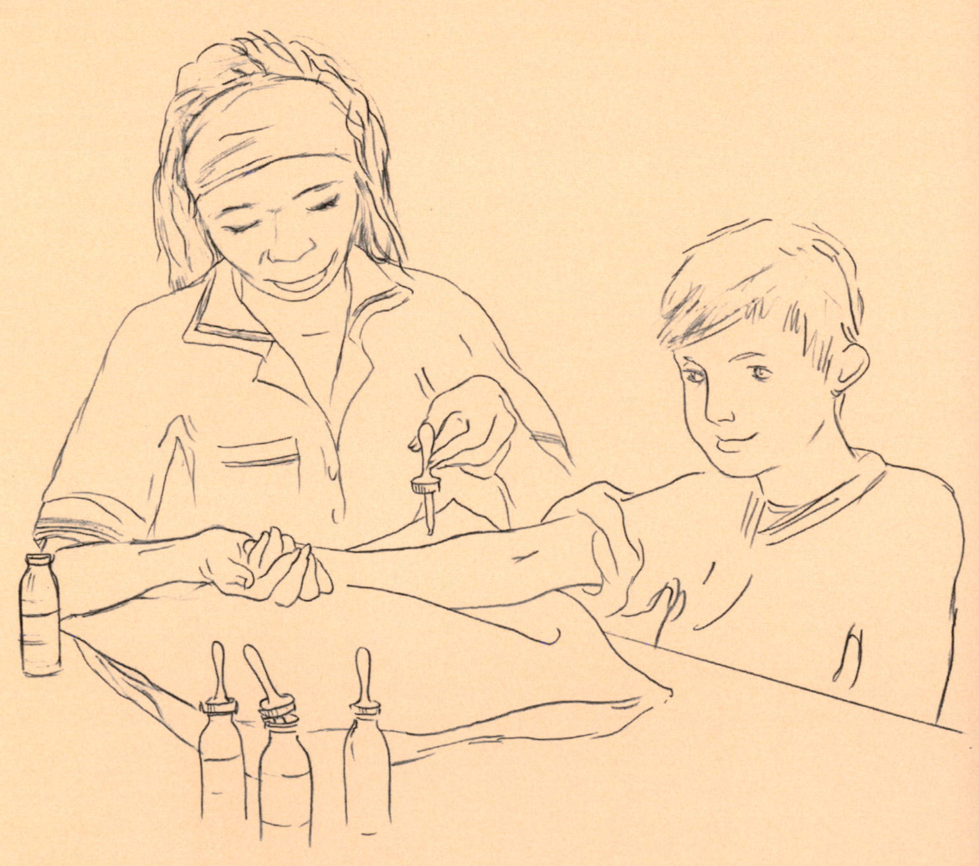

Allergy tests are a diagnostic tool doctors can use to determine the probability that an allergen is the cause of the problems. On their own, they cannot indicate how allergic someone is but they help doctors to build up a picture of a person's allergies. The tests are safe and non-invasive.

The two most commonly used are the skin-prick test and specific IgE blood tests (usually referred to as RAST, short for Radioallergosorbent Test). The purpose of these tests is to confirm which foods your child is allergic to. The specialist will choose the most appropriate test for your child and sometimes both will be used.

An accurate diagnosis relies on an interpretation of the test results *in conjunction* with a thorough examination of your child's health and previous allergic symptoms. Therefore your first consultation will involve a detailed assessment of your child's allergic history that will take up to 40 minutes. Testing and assessment can then take up to an hour. Below is a detailed description of what these tests involve and how to prepare for them.

Skin-prick testing

Skin-prick testing is the most common way to determine a child's allergens. It has the advantage of producing immediate results. The specialist will decide with you which allergens to test your child for.

What to expect

At the test, you will see a tray of small bottles of clear liquid containing purified extracts of the common allergens. You may be asked to bring along a sample of the food you suspect your child to be sensitive to. For example, Deborah takes along a small jar of honey to Thomas' appointments because it is an unusual allergen and would not be included in the standard testing kit at the hospital.

A drop of each allergen will be placed along the inside of your child's arm as well as a drop of histamine (positive control) that everybody should react to, and a drop of saline (negative control), which nobody should react to. If your child has severe eczema on both arms the specialist may test on his or her back instead.

The positive and negative controls are used to check that the immune system is responding normally. If your child does not react to the positive control, a normal reaction may be being hampered by the presence of antihistamines in the body. A reaction to the negative control indicates that the skin is hypersensitive and likely to react to anything placed on it – either situation would render the test invalid.

Each drop will be identified in pen and scratched into the skin with a prick-lancet (a thumb-nail-sized metal plate with a sharp nib at one end). Warn your child that they *might* feel a tiny scratch but reassure them it will be over quickly. Some children do cry, some barely notice the procedure and others watch with interest.

You will be asked to wait for about 15 minutes during which time any reaction to the substances will have occurred. To ensure an accurate reading it is important to be seen after the first ten minutes but before 20 minutes have elapsed. If you think you've been forgotten, go and find the nurse.

Your child's arm is going to itch. Try to discourage any scratching as this causes more redness and affects the result. Distract your child by playing a game or reading a book together.

We find that encouraging Zac to blow hard on the itchy bumps helps to put him off scratching at them. A packet of chewy sweets, that demands all his attention to get into, passes the time well too! Alice

The red swellings on your child's arm will be examined to find out which allergens he or she has reacted to. Each reaction will be measured in millimetres, using a plastic rule or the specialist's own judgement. Reactions can be anything from 1mm to several centimetres. Severe allergies can cause a red swelling that seems extremely large and can appear as soon as the substance is placed on the arm.

The specialist will interpret these results for you at the time and give you any guidance or prescriptions. Also see p.22 on allergy specialists.

Antihistamines

Your child's body will need to be completely free of antihistamine in order for skin-prick testing to give an accurate reading. The hospital should inform you how far ahead to stop giving your child antihistamine. If they haven't, ring up and ask for guidance *at least a month before* the appointment.

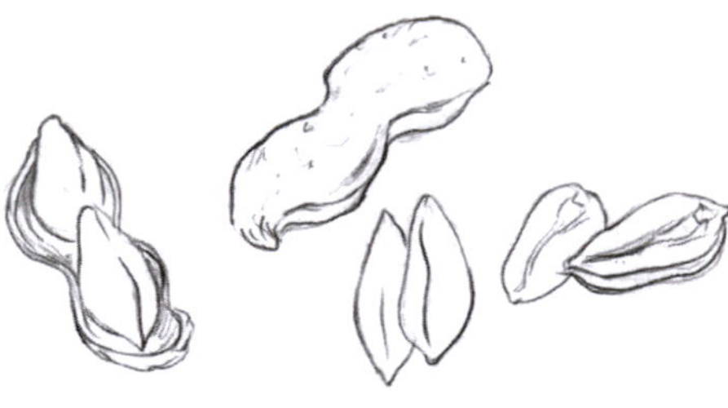

When we took Daisy to casualty with the peanut reaction they did say they could do tests in a controlled environment to find out how allergic she is and that we might have to carry around adrenaline pens if it was very severe but there was no referral or anything. Normally, I wouldn't just sit back and do nothing so I don't quite know why I haven't found out about it all, to be honest. I don't know if it's to do with not wanting to see her with needles and injections or that if I don't think about it I won't have to face up to it. Maybe what I've done is to convince myself that apart from the nut allergy everything else is just a mild inconvenience. The trouble is, I do still want to know. I just want the diagnosis over and done with – without actually having to go through it. Alison

RAST – Specific IgE blood testing

Testing blood for the level of antibody (IgE) it produces in response to specific allergens is commonly called RAST, short for Radioallergosorbent test. It is ideal for children who cannot come off their medication because it does not require the withdrawal of antihistamines.

The RAST test involves taking a sample of blood from your child's hand or arm with a syringe. A local anaesthetic, in the form of a cream, can be applied to the back of the hands or the crooks of the arms depending on where the nurse thinks the blood sample can most easily be drawn. Commonly known as 'magic cream' by the nurses, it takes about 40 minutes to become effective. There are cold spray anaesthetics which work immediately, and if you're lucky your hospital may have these, but be prepared to be told they don't.

Zac absolutely loved his first RAST test. We focused on the process and told him beforehand what to expect. So he was fascinated to see his blood zooming down the tube and into the little jar. We decided not to have the anaesthetic, which may have helped with the nerves as there was no waiting around. The needle is so thin and tiny I can't imagine you'd even feel it. We made the whole thing out to be really exciting, in a scientific sort of way, and he was captivated. Alice

As with all injections, occasionally children feel faint if they watch the procedure. Distraction is the key. Parents of small children have found that blowing bubbles does the trick while for older children, a sugar lollipop can work wonders.

Thomas has had a few RAST tests and at each one he has turned white and felt dizzy. This has got worse the older he's become and he has actually vomited and fainted at the sight of the needle. Last time I warned the nurse he was likely to faint so he lay down. It didn't stop him fainting, but at least I was prepared. Deborah

The blood sample will be sent to the laboratory for testing and the results usually take two to three weeks to arrive. Your child's specialist will interpret the results for you.

Interpreting test results

Skin-prick and RAST tests demonstrate the response of the immune system to specific substances. Your child's specialist will use the test results in conjunction with the medical history they took earlier to gauge the severity of your child's allergies and how best to manage them. Sadly, the specialist will never be able to give you a *definite* indication of whether your child will have an anaphylactic reaction but will prescribe your child adrenaline if they think there is any risk.

If you would like to read a detailed medical explanation of immune system responses and the role IgE antibodies play in allergy we recommend: *The Complete Guide to Food Allergy and Intolerance* and *The Allergy Bible* (Appendix).

Food challenges

A food challenge measures in real terms how much of their allergen a child can actually tolerate by feeding them increasing amounts, at regular intervals, and monitoring any reaction. Food challenges should only be carried out under medical supervision in controlled conditions, which means careful monitoring at every stage in an environment (usually a hospital) where all the necessary medication and resuscitation equipment is to hand. A successful food challenge will mean that you can confidently introduce the food into your child's diet.

Why are food challenges undertaken?

There are several indicators for using a food challenge in diagnosis:

- If skin-prick and RAST test results show a significant reduction in reaction from previous tests, the specialist may suspect that the food could now be eaten with no adverse reactions. In order to ascertain your child's actual tolerance of the food the specialist would use a food challenge.
- If your child's specialist is uncertain about the presence of a food allergy (following an inconclusive skin-prick and RAST for example) then a food challenge might be used to make an accurate diagnosis. If the food produces no reaction, other causes for your child's symptoms can be sought. If it does, the severity of the allergy can be measured and appropriate medication prescribed.
- The parents may have reason to believe that their son or daughter can now tolerate their allergen if, for example, their child has eaten it by mistake to no ill effect. In these circumstances both parents and doctor would want to find out if it really is safe to reintroduce that food into the child's diet.

What will happen at the food challenge?

Before the food challenge begins, the doctor or nurse will take a full medical history and obtain written parental consent. Your child will be weighed, have his or her lung function (peak flow), blood pressure, pulse rate and oxygen levels in the blood (SATS) measured and any marks or blotches on the skin noted. This will show your child's state of health prior to the challenge against which any changes that occur can be compared. Throughout the test physical signs will be carefully monitored and recorded.

Procedures vary slightly from clinic to clinic but most food challenges start with skin or lip contact, where the allergen is rubbed gently onto the skin or lips. A nurse will observe your child for at least 15 minutes for any reaction on the lips or face. If there is no reaction, the nurse will place a few millilitres in the mouth. Provided that there is no reaction at all they will repeat this at 20-30 minute intervals, increasing the amount until a normal portion for a child of that age is reached. You will be asked to wait in hospital for two hours after the last exposure, whether or not your child has reacted. Then you will be advised to monitor your child for 24 hours and reintroduce normal portions of the food into their diet. It is then important to keep intake regular, as with other foods they eat.

If *any* reaction occurs at any stage the food challenge will be stopped immediately and appropriate treatment given.

I took Thomas into hospital for a milk challenge. I expected that he might be sick at the tablespoon dose but wanted to prove that he would not have an anaphylactic reaction. But his mouth blistered and hives appeared on his chin when two millilitres of milk was put on his gum. The nurse immediately gave him antihistamine and Ventolin to prevent the reaction worsening. They told me he still reacts severely and is at risk of anaphylaxis. I was so disappointed but at least I now know where we stand. An 11-year-old boy in the ward managed the whole test without reacting whereas previously he reacted early on. That is encouraging and gives me hope. Deborah

How do I prepare my child for a food challenge?

Explain what is going to happen and why. Reassure your child that the challenge would not be done if it were unsafe; that although there might be an allergic reaction, the doctors and nurses will be on hand to treat it immediately; that your child is in safe hands; that you'll be there all the time; that this will help to find out whether your child will be able to eat this food from now on.

I took in some carrots for Zac's first challenge and the lovely Irish nurse looked me in the eye and said, 'Carrots are all very well but I think you could try some chocolate next time, don't you?' Alice

To undertake a food challenge, your child must be fit and well with no coughs or colds, and there must be no antihistamine in his or her system. Since these drugs can take from 48 hours to a month to clear, ring the hospital for advice well in advance. If your child is unwell or has to take antihistamine prior to the challenge you should arrange another appointment with the hospital.

A food challenge can take from a morning to a whole day to complete so take in a packed lunch and plenty of activities to keep you both occupied.

After Zac's successful peanut challenge, I was over the moon – I wanted to rush out and hug the world! We sat on the wall outside the hospital and ate ice creams, beaming from ear to ear. Alice

TOP TIP

If you feel that the unfamiliar and possibly frightening taste of the challenge food might upset your child, take in some of his or her favourite food to disguise it.

6 Emotional impact

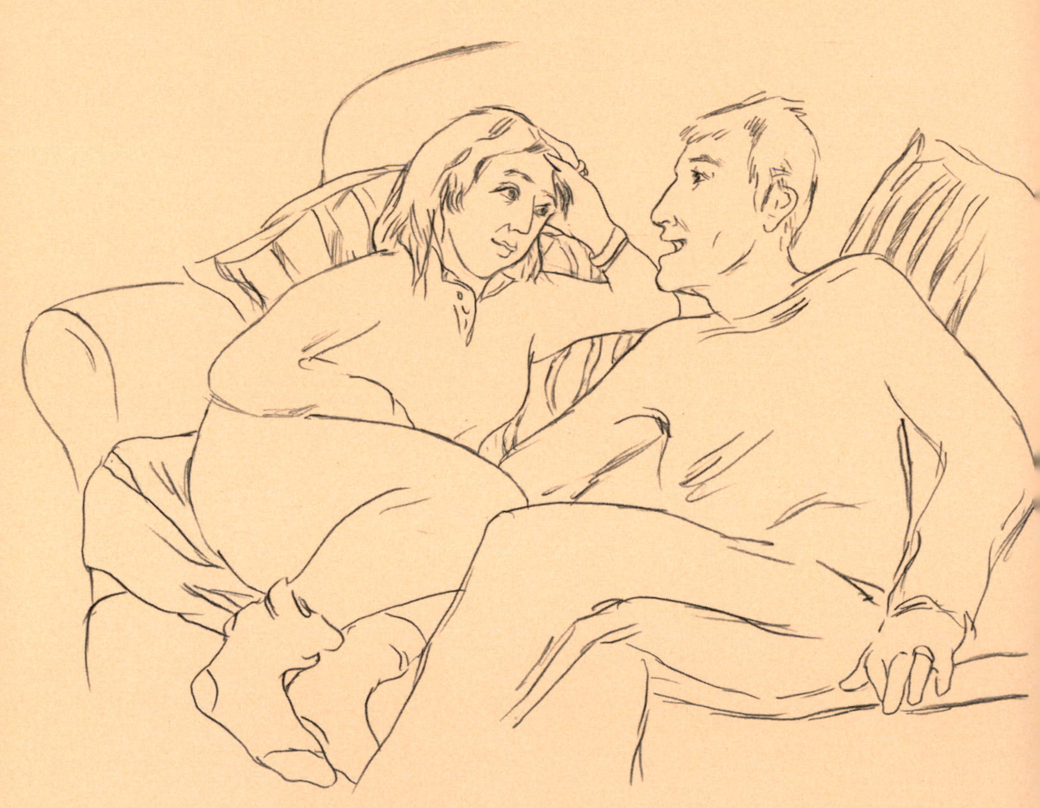

There is no right or wrong way to feel when your child is diagnosed with a food allergy. We all respond differently, depending on our own experience and expectations, how informed we are and how well we feel our child is being cared for by the medical professionals. The physical experience of allergy belongs to our child but as parents, we feel the emotional impact more significantly. The practical matter of caring for them falls to us and our emotional state may be reflected in how we adjust to those challenges.

Facing your fears

If it was just a case of, 'If Daisy has a glass of milk, she's sick everywhere' and that's all it will ever be, fine. I can live with that – it's inconvenient but not life-threatening. With anaphylaxis I just feel like it's a whole different thing. Alison

Having an anaphylactic child takes the stress of living with allergy to the extreme. Anaphylaxis is a life-threatening condition. Our children's safety is literally in our hands. That is scary.

All parents have fears about the safety of their children. I felt that what set me apart from other parents was that I was the one who was likely to give my son the fatal spoonful or sip. THAT responsibility was so heavy. Alice

We all worry about whether we would know what to do if our child did have an anaphylactic reaction. Would we act fast enough? Would we even be there?

Q: *My child has never had an anaphylactic reaction but I have been told that he is at risk and worry that I won't recognise a severe reaction in time.*

A: This is a common anxiety because we have all been told that giving adrenaline promptly is vital. To reassure you, the consensus among the parents we interviewed was that you will recognise an anaphylactic reaction. In fact, because you are aware of the possibility of a severe allergic reaction, you are more likely to overreact and give the adrenaline unnecessarily. If you are not sure, the general advice is that it is better to give the adrenaline than not, then call an ambulance and go straight to hospital. Be as well informed as you can and make sure that wherever your child goes, the adrenaline auto-injectors go too.

Fortunately, it is extremely rare for children to die from food-induced anaphylaxis. Research into the reasons why young children have died from anaphylaxis concludes that a failure to recognise how severe the reactions were and to give adrenaline straight away increases the risk of a fatal outcome.[3] Constantly being aware and reacting quickly is undoubtedly a vital factor in keeping your child safe. The fact that you are finding out more about how to care for your anaphylactic child means you are already minimising that risk.

Fatal and near-fatal reactions in children happen most often when:

- They or their carers are not carrying adrenaline auto-injectors.
- There is only one adrenaline auto-injector available and a second dose of adrenaline is required.
- The child's health is compromised by poorly managed asthma[4] or infection.
- The child has had previous severe allergic reactions.

***Always* carry two adrenaline auto-injectors and know how to use them.**

Although the threat of a serious allergic reaction is always there, we do adjust to living with it over time. The parents we interviewed all said that time and experience gave them the confidence to put allergy to the back of their minds and get on with living.

We all have nightmares

You are not alone if you lie awake in bed at night imagining situations that might put your allergic child in danger. Parents of allergic children have to live with tension. The key is to manage it well by building good habits:

- Keep adrenaline auto-injectors in one place in the home.
- Know where they are.
- Make it a habit to pick them up whenever you grab your house keys to go out.
- Carry a charged mobile phone with you at all times.

Many parents of allergic children register their details with Medic Alert (Appendix). Your child can wear a Medic Alert bracelet which bears a brief description of their medical details. Hospital staff can then telephone the organisation for further details. You should carry your child's medical card in your purse or wallet – clearly marking that these are your child's details and not your own. You can make your own version of the medical card if you have not joined Medic Alert but we strongly recommend that you make use of this internationally recognised service.

TOP TIP

Other parents say that with time, the anxiety becomes manageable. We can all be forgetful and find ourselves caught out for some reason or other, but we build good habits.

Showing affection

Giving your child kisses and cuddles is a natural and necessary part of their upbringing. However, once a food allergy has been identified, you are faced with having to be aware of everything that you have recently eaten, drunk or touched. Allergens passed from the lips or hands commonly cause an allergic reaction. Fortunately, these reactions are rarely severe, but even giving your child a red, blotchy face is upsetting.

In the early days, the sense of panic I used to feel when enchanted strangers leant into the pushchair to touch Zac's cheek was out of control. I was paranoid about what they might have just touched or eaten. I knew my protectiveness was completely over the top but couldn't help myself. It soon wore off, thank goodness.
Alice

You may also be worried when grandparents or friends, for example, play with your child. It's worth explaining to them why you're tense but try to keep a sense of perspective. Play and affection are vital for children. Learning to be comfortable with the risk of contact reactions is part of adjusting to life with an allergic child.

Supporting your partner

Isn't this just the hardest area when you're both stressed? How many of us are aware that our partner is getting sidelined in all the turmoil but can't seem to connect? When one parent spends a lot of time caring for the allergic child it is easy for the other to feel excluded.

Sometimes the parent who does most of the work and the worrying resents the fact that the other parent seems to carry little of the burden. It is so important to talk to each other about these feelings. It could be that the parent who is doing less actually feels the same stress but is in awe of the other's ability to cope and the level of competence shown.

It sounds obvious, but not taking your partner's support for granted and finding ways to share your stress is vital.

Reactions to stress

Finding out that you have severe food allergy in a family can make you feel scared, fearful, angry, guilty, anxious, in denial, hopeless, restless, even numb. Hopefully, you will also feel motivated to find out about overcoming the practical challenges of allergy. Duncan and Deborah explain how this can feel:

I don't know if I'm unusual, but I know my wife felt I opted out when Thomas' allergies were diagnosed. I certainly didn't mean to. I love my family dearly and would do anything for them. I think what happened was this: early on my wife got very involved in finding out all about allergies and got quite knowledgeable. I just felt numb. Her research and care for our child was wonderful, and I suppose my reaction was to leave things to her to sort out. She got on and did things. I just felt ignorant, so backed off all the more. I knew our son was being looked after wonderfully, but I didn't think enough about how lonely my wife felt. This caused a lot of stress between us as partners. I discovered later that she truly believed I didn't care.

I thought, 'She's doing a brilliant job – therefore she's coping'. I felt useless and I certainly didn't want to add to her hassles by talking about my own fear. Duncan

I did like to be the one in control of the situation and could never have let my husband be the main carer but some support would have been nice. The strain of eczema and asthma on top of Thomas' other allergies was what made my life almost unbearable.

I became completely caught up in caring for Thomas and abandoned my husband and our relationship. I saw him as lazy and uncaring. I thought he was backing away when I had built a barrier too. It only seemed to be at times when it all got too much and I broke down that I let him in. Both of our reactions made for a very difficult time. Deborah

Different roles

In most families, it is likely that the primary carer will become the most knowledgeable and that the other parent will rely on him or her for guidance and information.

Although I trust my husband to care for Daisy, I don't think he's as focused as me on what she should or shouldn't eat. If ever there was an accident I would feel that there was a much higher probability of it being with him than with me. It's not that he doesn't take it seriously but he hasn't been here all the time like me. I think he's a little bit complacent at times. He says things like, 'Oh she'll be alright, she'll be alright'. But you just don't take the risk. He wasn't here when I had to take her to the hospital, he met us there. When he does look after her on his own I leave out what she can have. He's one of those people who, if I'm prepared to take on the responsibility and the burden, will take a back seat. Alison

The primary carer is likely to be in the frontline of practical care 24 hours a day, unable ever to hand responsibility over entirely to someone else. This is hugely stressful, especially if the other parent is thought to be taking less responsibility. Although it is unrealistic to expect that both parents' roles could be the same, recognising the differences is an important step in offering emotional support to each other.

Early on, I would force-feed my husband information, things I'd found out, and was aware that often he didn't know what to make of it all. He was busy going out to work, he wasn't there at mealtimes. Also, while I was breastfeeding I had to change my diet – he didn't. I was the one shopping, cooking, working out on my own what Zac could and couldn't eat. So there was more immediate impact for me; he was distanced from it all. It annoyed me sometimes that he would seem to be checking everything with me – whether a certain cereal was suitable for Zac for example – and I felt like saying, 'Read the label. Don't ask me.' Of course, there were so many things he did have to check with me that it just became a habit and to be honest I'm glad that he kept checking rather than making a mistake. I think I must have been very bad tempered for a while, difficult to approach. On the plus side, he always listened and I was able to offload some of my anxiety that way. So, although he often didn't know how to help, he did without realising. Alice

Communication is the key: by voicing your feelings you can work together to conquer the initial complexities of having an allergic child.

TOP TIP

Communication

Communication is the key to supporting each other. However, problems with communication can be caused by many things. Unfortunately, the usual demands of family life do not stop while you concentrate on learning to cope with allergy. On top of this you may be battling tiredness, work and other ongoing responsibilities – or even depression.

We're not great at communication in this house! I got very frustrated to start with when my husband didn't seem that interested in the allergy and didn't read up as much about everything as I did, when I thought he should. I guess it was more difficult for him to be or feel involved as he wasn't there for the really bad reaction, nor at any of the appointments with the consultant or allergy clinics, but I would rather he'd gone to town on the internet like I did rather than having it relayed to him. Tracy

Despite all you are coping with, try to make space just for each other. Spend an evening without television; go out walking together; share a meal together; find an opportunity to talk. Be as honest as you are able. Be open about your differences. Perhaps keeping a diary or writing a letter to your partner would help you to communicate how you feel. Whatever you do, do not allow resentment to build up. Your children will benefit enormously from seeing parents who work together in times of stress.

We have been very supportive of each other and have found we cope with the situation in similar ways. My wife, Lilly, has been extremely strong in taking the brunt of the issues. Together, we have tried to make Lorie's life as normal as possible. Initially we both felt quite stressed and felt sorry for Lorie. We are much more relaxed nowadays and have learnt to accept the fact that she may never grow out of the allergies. Tom

Support from family and friends

Expect differing reactions from family and friends when you tell them that your child is seriously allergic. Some will be fantastic and offer you exactly the support you need. Some will long to make you feel better, reassuring you that it isn't as bad as it seems. Others will try to find answers to the problems and give you advice, whether you want it or not! Surprisingly, a few will leave you wondering if they have even heard at all.

Nowadays, I hear my family explaining Zac's allergy to people in terms that are accurate and forceful. However, there was a time when I wondered if they really understood me when I said that this could kill him. They didn't seem to understand how serious it was. I was still partly in denial myself but certain of one thing – I had to face the fact that this was dangerous and wasn't going to go away.

This struggle to make other people who love you understand the seriousness of anaphylaxis, when you are still trying to come to terms with what it means yourself, is hard. Because my family didn't want to see me so upset they kept ringing to tell me that so-and-so said lots of children were allergic to egg and grew out of it, or that a vaccine for hay fever had been found and surely this new discovery would help Zac eventually too. They meant well, but what I needed most at that time was for them to be supportive, to listen and offer practical help with looking after Zac while I figured out what to do next. Of course I didn't manage to say so at the time and it led to some strained relationships for a while. How pointless that seems, looking back.

My advice is to ask your family and friends for the support you need: 'Please come and stay for a few days, I need some help' or, 'Can you just listen while I tell you all this stuff that's floating about in my head without saying, "He'll probably grow out of it, dear"?' You could even write to them so they can read and reread what you're telling them. Alice

Telling family and friends was very difficult in the beginning. We wanted so much to be able to share our feelings with our family but found it increasingly frustrating that they didn't understand what we were telling them. Dawn

Persevere with those who have not yet understood the impact allergy is having on your life. Let them know how it affects *your* family. This is a new experience for most people and everybody needs to start somewhere.

When it came to telling friends and family about Peter's allergies we decided to just tell it as it was. Some of them are brilliant and we trust them to look after Peter but others are not. The thing that has caused us stress is other people's attitudes and levels of incompetence. We cope by taking the approach that food isn't the be-all and end-all of life which helps put things into perspective – Peter is a healthy, happy child and his allergy is not serious enough to impact too much on life. Angela

Taking a very direct approach can work well. Watch out though, even when you think friends have grasped it, they can still surprise you.

My friends have been great, very supportive. There's only been one incident when I went to have my hair cut and my friend looked after Daisy. I could see she had a walnut cake out on the side and I thought I can't leave without saying, 'Please make sure that Daisy doesn't get anywhere near it.' It was for the other mums who were coming round, not the children, but I felt I couldn't go without saying something. If that was me looking after somebody's child who I knew had a nut allergy I wouldn't even have brought it into the house, let alone put it out for the mums. My friend was fine about it: 'Of course I won't let Daisy near it.' But it would have made me feel more comfortable if she hadn't had it. Alison

Awkward situations like this can make you feel like a fussy over-protective parent, added to which there is the concern that when a friend is helping out, the last thing you want to do is cause offence by dashing round the house checking for potential dangers. Making a fuss is a necessary part of parenting allergic children and can have unexpected advantages.

I find that sometimes there's a silver lining. For example, when I say to my friends that Matthew can't eat this or that they feel easier about saying, 'Well we prefer not to eat such and such because of our religion.' Gwyneth

TOP TIP

Do remember to tell family and friends how grateful you are for their support. Help those who are willing to learn to care for your child (p.126). Give your family and friends a chance – they need time to adjust and learn – just like you.

Most importantly, go easy on yourself. So what if you snap at a loved one, storm about in tears, clam up and won't communicate for days? It happens. They'll forgive you. Forgive yourself.

Does anyone understand?

Although allergy is becoming more common and better publicised, you are still likely to find yourself in the minority amongst your close circle of friends. Bringing up an allergic child can be a lonely business.

I would have loved to have contact with another parent going through, or that had gone through, what I was facing. I did eventually get a contact number for another parent. It's so good to know they're there to chat to when you need them. Dawn

In the early days I just wanted there to be more publicity about allergy to help others understand. The press and TV coverage is better now but tends to focus on nut allergy. Many people think you're just a crank if you say your child has an allergy to milk or egg – they don't realise milk and eggs can be allergens too. Angela

When Zac was diagnosed I had no friends with allergic children, no-one to share my experience with. I found that my choices about where we socialised, what I fed him or where to send him to pre-school were based on completely different criteria from theirs. It set me apart in a small but significant way. Luckily I'm pretty independent, but I still missed being able to share the same concerns and gossip as my peers. Alice

It is especially frustrating as a parent when others confuse a serious food allergy with food intolerance.

When Thomas was eating his own special food at a Christmas party another mother asked me why. I told her he was allergic to milk, egg and nuts and she said her son was allergic to milk too. I thought I'd found a sympathetic mother in the same position but when she pointed out her son to me I saw he was happily eating chocolates and ice cream. She had no idea. Deborah

Bringing up an allergic child can be stressful and lonely. Our emotional response is influenced by the compassion, understanding and support of our doctors, friends, family and partners. Certainly those who feel well supported cope the best. Our hope is that the shared experiences in this book will empower you to tackle confidently the issues you are facing. You are not alone.

Thomas' story

by Debbie Carter

Thomas was a large (10lb 7oz) baby at birth. He made a strange noise as he breathed which meant he was labelled a 'grunty' baby but he was otherwise presumed healthy. Because he was a big baby a midwife convinced me to give him a bottle of formula whilst he was in hospital to stop him getting too hungry. Despite successful breastfeeding from the start I didn't think to question her.

We came home and I continued breastfeeding until I had cause to give him another bottle when he was three weeks old. All was fine until one o'clock in the morning when Thomas made a strange choking, strangulated noise and stopped breathing. Both my husband and I were immediately at his side, realising from sleep how quickly we had to act. After lifting Thomas and banging him on the back he spluttered and started breathing again. He was admitted to hospital the next day for various tests including a chest x-ray which showed some fluid on his lungs and early signs of asthma.

Over the next few months Thomas started vomiting thick, sticky mucus; passing green, foul smelling, thick stools full of mucus; breathing with difficulty (the skin on his ribs was being sucked in with each breath) and he had eczema all over his body. His lips, fingers and toes had a blue tinge and he had a generally 'wasted' appearance.

When Thomas was four months old we were told he needed to be tested for cystic fibrosis. His symptoms certainly matched the books I read about this disease but thankfully the tests proved negative. I continued my quest to discover what was wrong with Thomas until I read a book called *Asthma and Beyond* by Paul Sherwood, which contained these words: 'Cow's milk allergy can sometimes mimic the symptoms of cystic fibrosis'. I stopped all cow's milk products in his diet and there was a definite improvement in all the symptoms but it was not until I stopped breastfeeding that Thomas began to improve vastly. He was so highly allergic that the traces of cow's milk protein in my breast milk had been affecting him. Thomas was put on soya formula but, as is sometimes the case, he developed an allergy to soya too. He was then prescribed a special, prescription formula called 'PeptiJunior'. This is when the struggle to discover what Thomas could and could not eat began.

During the next year, feeding Thomas was generally a case of trial and error. We were prescribed adrenaline and lots of Phenergan (antihistamine) then sent away to get on with it! At the age of one, Thomas was on a restricted diet of Weetabix, bananas, chicken, potatoes and vegetables. We were extremely limited in where we could let him play and ended up staying at home to avoid the stress. Thomas had to learn quickly that although other children were eating ice cream, chocolate, sweets and cakes he had to stick to his breadsticks and bananas.

Despite a fairly bland diet Thomas developed severe eczema all over his body and face. He would scratch and rub himself on his sheets or the carpets to try to relieve the itching. His skin was constantly weeping and bleeding as if a big pan of boiling water had been thrown over him. At 13 months he was admitted to hospital to try to control his eczema and to give some relief to all of us. He was given his own room because of the danger from other children's snacks and drinks.

Wet-wrapping was a new practice for eczema at this stage and the nurses took it in turns practising the technique on him. It was not altogether successful and we were given an appointment for skin-prick testing. It was a struggle to find space on his body for the tests amongst all the eczema but they managed to do it on his back. These produced positive results to milk, egg, soya and peanuts.

At 15 months Thomas managed to climb up and get his sister Sarah's cup of milk and drink a little bit of it. I rushed in to find him looking red, puffy and covered in urticaria. His eyes began to roll, his face went sheet white, his lips blue and I knew that this was anaphylaxis. I gave him the adrenaline which stopped the eye-rolling and brought colour back to his face and lips. I was about to get in the car and take him to hospital when he started vomiting profusely. Instead I rushed back in and called 999. They were fantastic. The operator stayed on the phone, reassuring me and asking questions. I was terribly shaky and desperate to stop the chit-chat and tell her where to send the ambulance but was told it was already coming and that they knew where I was phoning from. She stayed on the phone until the ambulance arrived and the paramedic took over. We were taken to the hospital. Thomas was very pale and quiet for a long time afterwards but was fine. Two months later a similar thing happened when his sister Sarah (then aged three) gave him a bite of cheese 'to see if he's alright now'. It was after these two episodes that I realised exactly what we were up against.

It was at this time that Thomas' asthma took off with such intensity (and for no obvious reason) that he often needed a trip to casualty to use a nebuliser. We were visiting casualty so often that we bought a nebuliser to use at home to save the trauma of rushing off in the car with a sick child at all hours of the day and night. It was difficult to know what to do with him, apart from pumping him full of the drugs. I hated doing that, but we were helpless to do anything else. However, despite everything, by the time Thomas was two, he was managing a much more varied diet, although milk, egg, nuts, soya and all the derivatives of these remained firmly out of the question.

Then, when he was 25 months old, Thomas suffered another anaphylactic reaction – this time to honey. He also reacted one week later although we have never worked out what to. He was once more admitted to hospital. As well as the anaphylactic episodes, Thomas was suffering many less dangerous allergic reactions which we were able to treat with Phenergan; the asthma was still not under control and the eczema was grossly infected with staphylococcus. It was all clearly too much for his system and he became very unwell.

Whilst in hospital, Thomas had some kind of blackout with eye-rolling, marked pallor and blueness of the lips and skin. Doctors and nurses came rushing from all over the hospital as he lapsed into a deep unconscious state for two hours. He then came round and recovered completely. The reasons for this episode were a mystery but perhaps there is only so much a two-year-old can take and he had had enough.

He was by now at his most sensitive and was reacting to many things (though not with anaphylaxis). He also became allergic to his medicines – Phenergan, a calcium supplement and the Becotide inhaler. We went on holiday to Wales with strict instructions from our doctors to come home should he deteriorate – we were not to see a local doctor whilst away because of the fears that they would not be able to treat him effectively. On this holiday, Thomas suffered constantly. The sea water and sand stung his eczema; leaves in the forest caused urticaria and breathing problems, as did dog hairs on a steam train. He was awake every night, scratching in agony and terribly upset. We returned home with a very quiet, pale child. The local doctors knew they could do no more and had him admitted as an emergency to Southampton General Hospital under the care of Professor Warner and his team – world experts in the field of allergy.

Thomas underwent more tests including blood tests, skin-prick and ECG. It was discovered that the allergy level in his blood (IgE), which should have been 200 was raised to 1800. His food allergies were identified as cow's milk, egg white, egg yolk, peanuts and honey (all of which could cause anaphylaxis). His other allergies were identified as: dogs, cats, rabbits and all other furred animals, feathers, moulds and house dust mite (all of which cause asthma, urticaria and exacerbation of eczema). To help control this hyper-allergic state Thomas was prescribed Cetirizine, Cimetidine, Floxapen and Flixotide. Thomas' condition rapidly improved and he was able to return home with restored energy and zest for life just one week after being admitted.

Since this time there have been no further anaphylactic reactions. When he was three, we successfully reintroduced soya into his diet. The asthma has probably been the most difficult aspect with many trips to hospital over the years. His eczema has virtually disappeared. At six, after food challenges in hospital, Thomas' allergies to peanuts and well cooked egg were found no longer to be a problem. However, a milk challenge at nine gave an immediate reaction and we were told this allergy would probably stay with him throughout his life. But amazingly a further milk challenge at age 11 following a diminished skin prick reaction proved the experts wrong and Thomas is now completely free of his milk allergy as well. I cannot begin to describe the change to life this has caused or the feelings of utter ecstasy. It is unbelievable. We – and Thomas especially – have been through quite an ordeal as a result of allergies but, despite Thomas being at the extreme end of the spectrum, he has also shown that it need not be a lifelong sentence.

LET'S GET PRACTICAL

7 Feeding your baby

This chapter has been written in collaboration with leading allergy dietitian Kate Grimshaw.

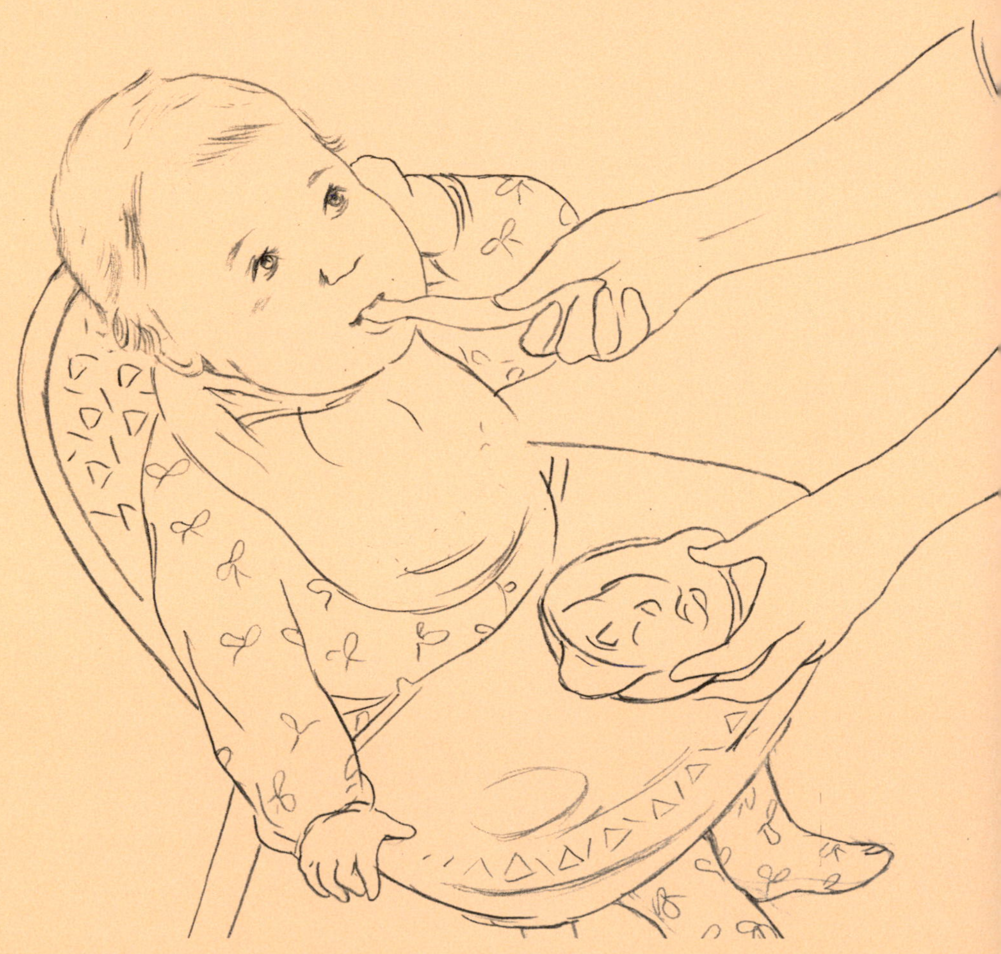

Breastfeeding

If your baby is atopic, don't be in too much of a hurry to get him or her onto solids and off the breast. You'll find the pressure to start solids before six months enormous, despite the fact that the World Health Organisation and Department of Health recommend that all babies should be breastfed exclusively for the first six months.[5] Waiting until six months to start weaning gives your baby's digestive and immune systems longer to mature so that they are better able to cope with food.

If breastfeeding is going well and your baby is gaining weight, there is no reason to feel pressurised into weaning before you and your baby are ready. However, it is important not to delay the introduction of solids beyond six months for developmental reasons. Remember, you can introduce solids and continue to breastfeed.

Breastfeeding is important for all infants, including those from allergic families, because not only is breast milk easily digested, but the mother passes on valuable antibodies to her baby. However, the breastfeeding mother with an atopic baby faces a cruel dilemma as it is also known that food proteins can be passed through breast milk in sufficient quantities to cause mild allergic reactions including rashes, diarrhoea, eczema, vomiting and colic.

Current advice is that breastfeeding remains the very best thing you can do for your atopic baby – just be alert to the possible problems and follow up any concerns promptly with your doctor. See *Allergic to breast milk* below.

Exclusive breastfeeding

Exclusive breastfeeding means just that – no bottles of formula (not even one), no bread sticks, no tastes of yoghurt – in other words nothing else passes the baby's lips except breast milk.

Exclusive breastfeeding will not guarantee that your child does not develop eczema, asthma or other allergies because some babies' genetic predisposition towards allergy is so strong, but it will give him or her the best chance there is.

Allergic to breast milk

There are rare cases where babies are allergic to something in their mother's breast milk. In this case you may need to exclude the suspected food/s from your diet or the doctor will recommend that you stop breastfeeding and will prescribe a hydrolysed formula. A hydrolysate has undergone a process to break down the proteins so that it has a significantly reduced allergic potential and, in most cases, does not cause a reaction even in highly sensitised babies. If this is your situation, you will be under careful medical guidance.

If it is recommended that you go on an exclusion diet yourself and continue to breastfeed, you should be given advice on how to do this by a dietitian to ensure that your diet is nutritionally adequate. Cutting foods out of your diet is difficult, so do not feel forced to do this if it is too much for you. It is a way to continue breastfeeding, if that is what you wish.

If it is thought best that you stop breastfeeding it can be a very emotional time, particularly if you had planned to breastfeed for a long time. If you are going to stop breastfeeding, you will need to reduce your milk supply gradually, so make sure you seek qualified advice on how to do this – the last thing you need is a bout of mastitis. You may also be coming to terms with a mix of emotions about giving up breastfeeding.

Impossible as it sounds, try to take time out to refresh yourself and rest so that you can keep all this in perspective. It's easy to underestimate the psychological impact of what you are going through. Many hospitals have their own breastfeeding supporter, a midwife who specialises in helping breastfeeding mothers. Help is also available from your local NCT breastfeeding counsellor or La Leche League representative (Appendix). Both organisations provide free support and counselling to all mothers. Contact your health visitor for support. She may also be able to arrange for some help in the home if you need practical assistance. Make sure you let your family and close friends know what is going on and ask for help and support.

Supplementary formula feeds in maternity wards

If you know in advance that you want to breastfeed your baby, beware of supplementary bottles of formula milk being given on the maternity ward.

The midwives force-fed Peter formula at birth when he refused to feed from me. I was furious and wonder if this has contributed to his problems. Angela

Angela wanted to breastfeed Peter (who is allergic to egg and milk products) and could have done with better breastfeeding support rather than the option she least wanted, formula milk.

You may need to work hard to help staff understand just how important it is to you that your baby is not given formula milk. Explain that you have allergies in the family and inform each new shift of midwives if necessary. Some mothers have put a notice on the baby's crib stating: 'NO FORMULA, BREAST MILK ONLY'. You may still have to face pressure on the ward, but at least your baby won't be given formula milk without your consent or knowledge.

If there is a medical need for your child to be given an infant formula, then ask that they are given a formula that has proven reduced allergenicity, e.g. Nutramigen, Nan HA. These formula milks have been shown to reduce the risk of developing an allergy compared to feeding with a standard infant formula.

Breastfeeding and going back to work

For many breastfeeding mothers the switch to formula milk seems inevitable if they decide to go back to work. Be reassured though, for every mother who feels she has no choice, there is another mother pumping breast milk at work one day to leave for her baby the next.

I liked breastfeeding Daisy and didn't want to stop, so it was going against everything that I wanted really. Alison

A common method is to use a double breast-pump to express milk during the day, store the expressed bottles in the fridge at work in a cool-bag to give to the childminder the next morning, and so on. Take in a small bottle of washing-up liquid and a kitchen roll so you can wash and dry your pump hygienically. It is a good idea to have a supply of frozen breast milk at home as a back-up (for those days when you dash out of the office and leave the cool-bag behind).

An added advantage of expressing whilst at work is that your milk supply will not be interrupted, so there will be no disruption to feeds on the days when you're not working.

Further support and information is available from a variety of sources – your health visitor, the NCT Breastfeeding or La Leche League help lines.

Going back to work after having a baby is a big adjustment anyway and it is a common perception that expressing milk at work will be difficult or embarrassing. If you have an atopic baby though, it is well worth considering because the benefits are believed to be so great.

However, if you find the logistics of expressing milk impossible in your circumstances, you may be able to give a hydrolysed formula milk (p.66) for the day feeds and continue to breastfeed for the early morning, early evening and night feeds.

Bottle feeding

If you suspect that your baby might be allergic to formula, it is important to talk to a doctor about your concerns. The doctor will be able to tell you whether the symptoms could be due to allergy or have some other cause.

Your doctor may advise you to try a different formula milk. Do not expect immediate results as it can take from 24 hours to two weeks for a baby's symptoms to clear up but, if you see no improvement, go back to the doctor.

I thought I'd try Daisy with bottled milk but as soon as the milk hit her tummy she just brought the whole lot back up. I spent a fortune on different types of formula but everything just made her sick. I spoke to the health visitor who said, maybe she was milk intolerant. In the end we switched her to soya formula and she seemed fine on that. Alison

If the doctor prescribes a hydrolysed formula and your baby's symptoms improve, ask your doctor about testing the cow's milk formula again after a month. It may be that the improvement was due to a coincidental recovery or that lactose intolerance has been cured by a month's avoidance and your baby will be able to go back onto cow's milk formula. However, if your baby's symptoms were severe and involved any swelling around the lips and mouth, any reintroduction should be done under medical supervision.

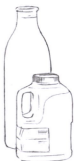

Formula milk is made from cow's milk

This may seem like an obvious statement but it is surprising how many parents don't know that a bottle of formula milk is an introduction of cow's milk, the most common allergen among babies. Mixing up baby rice with formula milk, giving the odd bottle here and there or bottle feeding exclusively all mean that you are feeding your baby cow's milk.

Soya formula not recommended

Soya formula is no longer recommended by the Department of Health for any baby under six months of age[6] and should ideally not be given below the age of a year due to phyto-oestrogens in the milk. Also, many infants with a cow's milk allergy are also allergic to soya so it is not considered sensible to give soya milk to children who are or who have a suspected milk allergy. Unfortunately, parents of allergic babies are still being advised to switch to soya formula by some doctors and health visitors. Although it can bring a short-term improvement in symptoms, the long term implications for atopic babies are not good because they may well become sensitised to soya as a result.

Hydrolysate

If your baby is reacting adversely to cow's milk formula and you have reason to believe that allergy is the cause, ask your doctor to prescribe a hydrolysed formula. Hydrolysates contain modified milk protein and have significantly reduced allergic potential. Don't be pushed into using soya formula if you have reservations.

If your baby has *already* had a clear allergic reaction to cow's milk formula, the same applies: you should be prescribed one of the lower risk hydrolysate formulas, not soya. Only introduce dairy products later under careful medical supervision, in case your child has a more serious allergic reaction.

Lactose intolerance

Lactose is a sugar present in all human and animal milk. In simple terms, if a baby does not produce enough of an enzyme called lactase in their tummy to digest this sugar, they suffer abdominal pain, vomiting and diarrhoea as a result. This enzyme deficiency is not a common condition but infants can have a secondary lactose intolerance that may last a few months after a bout of gastroenteritis. Lactose intolerance is well understood by doctors and easily treated.

An allergy to cow's milk can be misdiagnosed as lactose intolerance, so if your baby's symptoms do not improve quickly, go back to your doctor. One of the reasons for this confusion is that diarrhoea (from gastroenteritis for example) often causes a temporary lactase deficiency in babies, so that tests for lactose intolerance produce a positive result, masking the underlying allergy.

Colic and cow's milk

Colic causes a baby to scream, often for hours at a time, and draw up its legs due to painful spasms in the tummy. Among the many theories on what causes this painful condition, there is growing evidence to suggest a link between sensitivity to cow's milk and colic. Although more common in formula-fed babies, it also applies to breastfed babies because cow's milk proteins can pass through the mother's milk in sufficient quantities to upset highly sensitive babies.

It might be worth bearing in mind that stimulants such as tea, coffee, alcohol and chocolate can also upset a baby's system, so you could try withdrawing them for a week to see if your baby's symptoms improve. Reintroducing them one at a time should help you pinpoint the culprit.

Let them eat mud pies

Let your babies and children get dirty. Let them eat mud pies. Sounds like a joke? It's not.

There are a number of current theories about the reasons for the increase in allergies over the last forty years. One such theory, the 'hygiene hypothesis', is concerned with the possible link between exposure to parasites and bacteria at an early age and the development of allergies. Allergy is far less common in poorer, subsistence cultures than in the sanitised, developed world.

This theory is relevant to food-allergic children because the very same mechanisms in the body's immune system that are designed to fight certain parasites and bacteria (IgE antibodies) are the ones implicated in food allergy. So perhaps if we were exposed, as nature intended, to more dirt and germs upon entering the world, we would be less allergic.

We are told repeatedly during pregnancy how important sterilisation and cleanliness is for the health of our babies. Much attention is given to bedtime routines including a soothing bath and we are led to believe that squeaky clean babies are a reflection of good mothering. While we quite rightly want to protect our children from toxoplasmosis or nasty stomach bugs, it seems a little bit of rolling in the mud is not such a bad idea.

In short, some researchers believe being too fastidious about hand washing, keeping your baby away from other children's germs or stopping them from crawling about and getting mucky in the garden is unhelpful when it comes to allergy. Try to strike a sensible balance between exposure and protection.

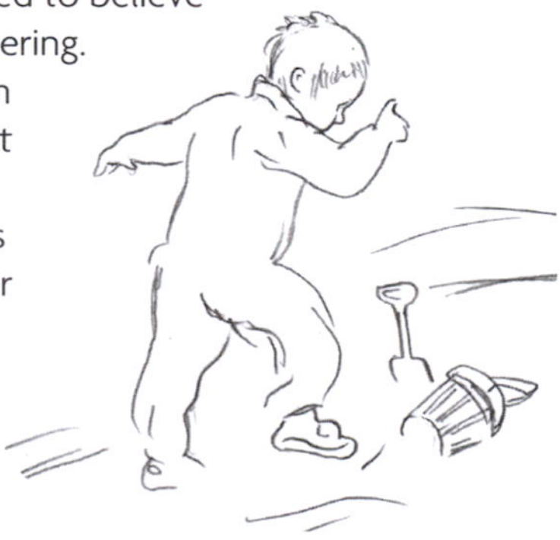

Weaning

Wean: to accustom an infant or other young mammal to food other than (esp. its mother's) milk.[7]

After six months, a baby has used up the iron stores accumulated whilst inside the womb. As there is no iron in breast milk or standard infant formula milk (although there is iron in follow-on formulas), and other nutrients are also needed, it is essential to begin weaning at six months or very soon after. Another reason not to delay introducing solids beyond six months is that there appears to be a window of opportunity for infants to learn how to deal with lumps, which seems to close at 10–11 months. If children have not experienced adequate lumps and texture by this time they will subsequently not readily take to lumps in their food. During weaning, babies get used to the taste of foods other than milk and their digestive systems gear up to extracting the nutrients they will need once they are fully weaned.

When I read 'allergic', it honestly didn't occur to me that my child might be more allergic than me. Alice

If baby-care books or weaning leaflets produced by food manufacturers mention allergy, the information is often slim. It might suggest avoiding certain foods 'if your child is likely to be allergic' or 'if there is a history of allergy in the family'. But how many of us find this advice too general to be of any practical use, or skim over this part assuming it won't apply to our baby? The shock of finding your baby is allergic to something you'd assumed was a safe, basic food can leave you feeling disillusioned.

We started weaning Lorie at four months but obviously we had no knowledge of her allergies at this stage. Once we were aware of her allergies we were given very little advice from anyone and struggled mostly on our own. Lilly

One of the key things that is missing for allergic families is the easy, carefree relationship with food enjoyed by other families. But don't worry – that enjoyment of food *can* come back into your lives and the following pages examine ways to make it possible. Embrace this new approach and start to enjoy food with your allergic child again.

How do I know if my baby will be allergic?

A history of allergy in the family means anything from having hay fever yourself, to a partner who had asthma as a child, a sister with a latex allergy or a brother who can't tolerate egg. It even includes a mother who is anaphylactic to bee stings or granny's eczema – so heed those allergy warnings, they do apply to you. Breastfeed exclusively and wean sensibly.

What sort of reaction should I be looking for?

Signs that your baby may be allergic to a food can be rashes (including nappy rash); loose, watery, offensive-smelling poo (or more rarely, persistent constipation); colic; a runny nose which doesn't appear to be a cold; a bloated tummy; vomiting; urticaria (nettle rash) anywhere on the body; and eczema. You may also see a strong, immediate reaction to the food such as swelling and redness of the lips, mouth and face or wheezing as soon as the food is eaten.

When I gave her scrambled egg, she went very, very quiet and within a minute of it all going down she was violently sick. She's had eggs since and she comes up in these red welts on her face as well and I notice that's definitely got worse. If you give her egg in cake she's fine, anything where the egg is diluted or broken down she's okay with as long as it's not too eggy. Alison

Allergic reactions to food occur the second time an allergen is encountered, not the first. Sometimes it may seem as though your baby is reacting to the first exposure but in fact this means that, whether you were aware of it or not, they have already encountered that food.

After we discovered Lorie's egg allergy, we became much more cautious about foods. We were advised to introduce new foods one at a time and we discovered that unfortunately Lorie had other food allergies like pea and lentil, which are legumes and related to peanuts. On these occasions she would be violently sick and her whole body came out in urticaria, making her distressed and very itchy. Lilly

Although some allergic reactions are immediate, it can take up to 72 hours for a reaction such as eczema to appear.

Conflicting advice

Weaning is an area of great interest for all parents, not just for those of allergic children or those considered to be at high risk. All parents want to do the best for their child and allergy parents are no different. The main concern for all parents is the same: 'What foods do I give and when and how much?'

Weaning guidelines come from all different sorts of places and no two are the same but they all tend to be prescriptive. Some people find this approach very helpful and if you choose a framework, stick to it, but remember that it is not the only way to do things and don't let following such a plan add to your anxiety. The stress over weaning is often increased by prescriptive guidelines but because that is how weaning information is *usually* presented we tend to think that is what we should be following.

Much as you may long for concrete guidance of the 'If you do this, your baby won't be allergic' variety, currently this information is not known and anything that promises this is misleading. Over the following pages you will find sensible guidelines for weaning, whether your child is allergic or at risk of being allergic.

Weaning Guidelines

In this section you will find the tools to make more liberated choices about the order in which you introduce foods to your child, confident in the knowledge that there is no evidence that delaying the introduction of a food beyond six months reduces the likelihood of a child reacting to it. This may be vastly different to the advice you are being given elsewhere because parents with allergic children are being advised to delay introducing potentially allergenic foods. Evidence emerging now indicates that there is no advantage in delayed weaning; in fact it may make matters worse. *Any* food (with the exception of nuts, seafood and honey) can be given after six months. Here we cover the principles of how best to introduce these foods.

Throughout weaning, introduce each new food in turn, working through foods one at a time so that if a reaction occurs you can readily identify the cause.

- Only introduce one new food each day.
- Give each new food for three days consecutively.
- Once a new food is introduced keep it in the diet regularly.

If your child has already been diagnosed with an allergy, exclude anything to which your child is already allergic and discuss the weaning programme with your child's dietitian. (See p.75 *Weaning a baby who has already had an allergic reaction.*)

First weaning foods

It is recommended that solids are not introduced until your child is six months old but certainly *never* before four months.[8] If you do introduce solids before six months just keep to the first weaning foods detailed in the table below.

Fruit	Apple, pear, banana, peach, nectarine, apricot, plum, mango, papaya, melon
Vegetable	Carrot, parsnip, potato, sweet potato, butternut squash (squashes), swede, turnip, celeriac, broccoli, cauliflower, courgette, onions, leeks, celery, fennel
Cereal products	Baby rice, pureed rice, oats

It is perfectly normal to introduce a food for the first time combined with another food that has been taken before, e.g. baby rice with banana, carrot with potato.

Follow on foods

Following on from these first weaning foods, you can now introduce all other foods with the exception of the few detailed below.

- Nuts: if there is allergy in the family it is recommended by the Department of Health that you do not give any nuts until the age of three.
- Seafood: not until over the age of one for food hygiene reasons, not because of allergy.
- Honey: not until over the age of one for food hygiene reasons, not because of allergy.

Using the same weaning principles of one new food at a time eaten over at least three consecutive days, increase the new foods in your baby's diet over the coming months and years. If you have any cause for concern that a food may be causing allergic symptoms in your child, remove the food from his or her diet and seek medical advice as soon as possible.

You *can* introduce new foods every day if they are essentially the same food – for example, milk one day followed the next by yoghurt, followed the next day by cheese and so on. All these food products are made from cow's milk and so you are not introducing a new food, just the same food in different forms.

TOP TIP

You may find it helpful to jot down the days you plan to try the new foods. This helps with shopping and food preparation. It can also help identify the culprit food if your child does have a reaction.

Theory and practice

The theory all sounds very neat, doesn't it? In practice, you'll find you have all sorts of questions as you go along. Ask your dietitian and allergy specialist for answers. It's only normal that the questions pop up when you're at home staring into the saucepan, not sitting in the waiting room, so don't feel silly.

Some common questions:

Q: *Peas, beans, lentils and pulses are from the same food group as peanuts. At what age should I introduce these vegetables?*

A: Although some children are known to react to these foods it is quite rare. There is no reason to delay the introduction of these foods beyond six months as there is no evidence that doing this reduces the likelihood of an allergy developing. They are a good alternative source of iron to red meat and also mash up well, so are a good way of introducing texture into your child's diet.

Q: *I've been told that strawberries are allergenic. When should I give them to my child? What about raspberries and blackberries? Should I start with cooked fruits, as in yoghurt, or fresh? So many baby yoghurts contain berries.*

A: Strawberries are able to release histamine directly, appearing to cause an allergic reaction particularly around the mouth where the juice comes into contact with skin that may often be sensitive. It is in fact not an allergic reaction but in some children with existing eczema eating strawberries can cause flaring. Consequently, there is no reason to delay the introduction of strawberries or other berries beyond six months.

Q: *I've heard that sesame is highly allergenic – should I be avoiding it too?*

A: More children are starting to react to sesame than in the past but, as with all other foods, there is no evidence that delaying the introduction of any allergic food beyond six months reduces the risk of an allergy to that food developing. Sesame is a good source of iron so should not be eliminated unnecessarily from the diet.

Q: *My son is allergic to dairy products and can't have normal yoghurts. Is it okay to wean on soya yoghurts and soya milk instead?*

A: Yes, so long as the child is over six months. Soya formula is no longer recommended for any baby under six months of age[9] and should ideally not be given below the age of a year due to phyto-oestrogens in the milk but giving some soya products as part of a balanced diet in weaning is fine.

Q: *Milk to drink or for cooking only? I've been told not to give milk as a drink until after one year – why is that and can it be given earlier?*

A: Milk can be given in cooking after six months of age but should not be given as a drink until one year of age because of its sodium (salt) content.

Q: *I have a daughter who is allergic to milk and nuts. Should I keep her new baby sister off milk to be on the safe side?*

A: No. Although your new daughter is more likely to have a food allergy because you already have one allergic child, there is no need to keep her off milk unnecessarily. Just introduce it after six months as an ingredient (e.g. a biscuit) first. If there is no reaction, introduce milk starting with small amounts first. The standard advice for nuts when there is allergy in the family is not to introduce them until the child is over three years of age.

Q: *My mother always says, 'Give them a little bit of what you're having, just mash it up'. Is this a good idea?*

A: For allergic children this may be the worst possible kind of advice, especially if you are unsure exactly what is in your food. So, pureeing up some of your home-made roast chicken, roast potato and plain boiled vegetables is a safe option but if you are having a pasta dish made with a 'cook-in-sauce' you should not give this to your child unless you know all the ingredients in the sauce (and the rest of the dish) and they have all been eaten previously without reaction. Only give your child what he or she has had before and one new food each day.

Q: *Does it matter whether I first give foods cooked or raw, when they are foods that can be eaten raw?*

A: For the main allergenic foods,(10) particularly egg, it is best to give them cooked first as an ingredient (for example, in cake). If there is no reaction to the cooked version it is safe to introduce it raw. For low allergenic foods, e.g. carrots and cucumber, you can introduce the food raw if you wish.

Q: *Can I give a new food cooked in a dish or cake, for example, or do I have to give it on its own?*

A: Yes, as long as your child has had all the other ingredients before.

Variety

Some allergists believe it may be best not to give your baby too much of the same foods every day because this could provoke sensitivity. This does not mean that you should panic if your baby eats toast at breakfast and bread at lunch; just don't give him or her bread, for example, at every meal, every day. This is a good weaning principle anyway as the ultimate aim is to make your child's diet as varied as possible.

Making life easier during weaning

- **Give new foods in the morning:** try out new foods in the morning or at lunchtime. This gives you plenty of time to see whether your child reacts.
- **Store small amounts:** cook enough food for two or three portions to minimise the time you spend cooking. Store unused portions in the fridge or freezer.
- **Make two lists:** stick two lists on your fridge – one for the foods you've yet to try and the other for foods you've already tried. As you work your way down the list, transfer each food across. This is not only encouraging but acts as a quick reference when you're too tired to think.
- **Don't get caught short:** keep well stocked with groceries. That way, you won't find yourself having to introduce something earlier than you wanted to.

Commercial baby foods

At some stage you may want to explore pre-packaged baby foods and there are more available for allergic babies than you might think. Once you've found the safe ones, they help remove the burden of cooking every meal from scratch.

There will always be a slight risk of contamination in commercial products and occasionally mislabelling occurs. When mistakes are discovered, manufacturers are quick to inform allergy organisations like the Anaphylaxis Campaign who send out alerts to their members. This is a very useful service. As a basic precaution, check that what is in the jar or packet looks and tastes like the description on the label.

How to choose from all the baby foods available

Generally the ingredients labelling on baby food is clearer and easier to understand since the new labelling laws that came into force in November 2005. However, do not make any assumptions about what is in a product by how it is described. Phrases such as, '*Suitable from 4 months*' and similar labels can be unhelpful. The '*Contains*' or '*Free from...*' boxes are much more helpful in quickly identifying which products should be suitable but really there is no getting away from the need to always read the list of ingredients.

TOP TIP

Do remember that, from time to time, companies change their recipes so always read ingredients labels. Manufacturers often highlight a change in ingredients by displaying *New Recipe* or *New and Improved* or something similar on the front of the packet.

Weaning a baby who has already had a serious allergic reaction

Weaning a baby who has already had a serious allergic reaction to food can be very stressful, the burden of which falls on the primary carer, usually mum. You may be on your own with your baby for most meals, added to which the responsibility of shopping and cooking falls to you. There are stages when every mouthful feels like a gamble. There is no way round this. .

I had found weaning my son confusing even before his allergic reaction, because everywhere I looked for guidance suggested a different set of foods. Once he'd had a bad reaction it became even more stressful, not least because I couldn't help feeling I'd been doing it all wrong. Why didn't I know then what I know now about weaning babies? I hadn't worked through foods systematically so I could easily identify a reaction. I wish I'd been smart enough to work out that all the weaning guidelines are different because there is no 'one and only' way to do it. Conflicting advice can become a trap – understanding the principles of weaning is so much more useful. Alice

The most sensible course of action in this situation is still to introduce new foods one at a time and start off with a small portion, e.g. half a teaspoon. Although the same principles of weaning apply, you may find you just feel more nervous about the whole process. However, once you are through it, life becomes so much easier because you know for sure what your baby can or can't eat. Your baby will have as balanced a diet as possible and you can gradually widen the range of foods within the limitations of his or her allergies.

Being frightened

After the traumatic experience of seeing your child suffer an allergic reaction, it's easy to regard every untested foodstuff as an 'enemy' but there really is no need. The whole point of a steady approach to weaning is that you test foods cautiously. If there is a food you are particularly nervous about wait for the weekend when other adults are around to share the load.

We are more fearful of trying new foods now, not just because of a potential anaphylactic reaction but because they might make Harvey's skin flare up and we will be up all night with him scratching and unable to sleep. His eczema and food reactions are always worse when he is ill or coming down with something, so he might react to something that is usually okay. Because the skin on his face is so sensitive when food gets on it, it can come up red and sore and then it's hard to tell whether he's having a reaction to food. It makes the whole weaning process more difficult. I have to admit that we sometimes stick with giving Harvey the same foods because we don't want his eczema to flare up or risk a more serious reaction. Sue

Try to remember that picking a good day to try a new food is more important than charging on with 'the plan'. An important element of this process is your own mental state. Anything which unduly upsets and panics you is not good for you or your baby.

If it's all getting too much, just coast for a while using the foods that you've already tried and tested. However, do not fall into the trap of holding back from introducing new foods into your child's diet once you have discovered a number of foods that are taken safely. If you do this you will end up with a child who has a very limited diet, not because of their allergy but because they have not encountered new foods and have become fussy. Make your ultimate goal being able to give your child as wide a diet as possible.

Weaning is more stressful if you know there's a chance your baby is going to react badly to foods, no doubt about it. For me it was important to remind myself that it wasn't my fault that my perfect, beautiful baby turned out to be allergic, that I was doing a good job and most importantly, what would be would be. Alice

Monitoring your baby's intake day in, day out is tedious and nerve-racking and if you are breastfeeding and having to restrict your own diet as well, you can easily become mentally and emotionally exhausted.

TOP TIP Give yourself a pat on the back for coping with twice as much as most other mothers and take each day as it comes.

You may find yourself keeping a record of which foods you give, when and how (p.77). Also read *Cooking: alternatives and adapting recipes* (p.92) to help you work round the limitations of a diet excluding certain foods.

Final word

As with other aspects of parenting, people always like to give you their opinion, whether you welcome it or not. Attitudes to weaning are no different. There are cultural and generational differences; there is professional advice and anecdotal evidence, and then your own preconceived ideas to take into account.

For your own peace of mind you must remember that there is *no* guaranteed way of preventing your child having a reaction to any food. Use this knowledge to liberate yourself from worrying about doing the wrong thing, to find your own way through and be happy with it.

A lot of research is being carried out to establish the best way to wean a child to reduce the likelihood of a food allergy developing. However, we currently do not know what that way is. Unfortunately, sometimes researchers talk about possible actions as if they are proven, causing confusion and conflicting advice. Those of us working in this field need to be more honest about what is 'known' and what is 'theorised' to help reduce the conflicting advice being given. Kate Grimshaw

Food and symptoms diary

In a food and symptoms diary you record the quantities and times of what your baby eats, including breastfeeds or formula milk, alongside a record of any symptoms, with time, duration and severity of each. The purpose of this is to enable you and your doctor to determine which foods are causing your baby's symptoms. Two or three weeks are usually sufficient to see patterns emerging.

In the very beginning we were advised to keep Jake off dairy, egg, nut, fish and wheat. We were able to reintroduce wheat after eight weeks to no ill effect. We were also advised to keep a food and symptoms diary which was a great help with introducing new foods. Fruit and vegetables are the first foods that many babies have and, on the whole, these were safe for Jake. Using the diary made introducing new foods easy, as we were able to keep a record of any reactions. Dawn

Keeping this detailed record is not necessary as a part of normal weaning but you may be advised by the doctor to start a food and symptoms diary if your baby appears to be reacting badly to food.

How to keep a food and symptoms diary

Use an exercise book and divide the pages into columns to keep an accurate record of what your child eats and when. If your child is having reactions to a number of foods and allergens, you will have to keep as detailed a picture as possible. You may find that more columns will make it easier to re-read later. Find a style that suits you. If you are breastfeeding, you may be asked to keep a record of your own food and drink intake too, because something you are eating could be passing through in the breast milk and causing the problem.

I kept our first food diary in an old school exercise book, dedicating a page to each day. One side of the page was for food and the other for symptoms. At the back of the book I glued in any labels rather than writing out all the ingredients. When Thomas was older, I was asked to keep a food diary for the dietitian to see if he was getting enough nutrients in his very basic diet. She wanted to know the amounts of each food he was eating which meant measuring and weighing – that was a pain! Deborah

I had a big office desk diary where I just wrote down everything Matthew ate. He was quite young so it really was simple. If it was a baby food jar I'd just take off the label and stick it in the book. I didn't keep a record of what I was eating but I was also writing down the state of his skin which was up and down. I could see no link at all between the foods and his eczema. Gwyneth

Example of a food and symptoms diary
A sample page taken from Zac's food and symptoms diary.

Time	Food & Drink	Notes, Symptoms & Medication
6.45am	Breast milk	
8am	Prune, Weetabix, Breast milk	Teething. Lots of dribbling
12noon	Toast, Lamb casserole Couscous, Olive oil Spinach, Apple	Not much appetite. Ate half More thirsty than usual. Hot? Extra water
5pm	Water biscuits Cheese sandwich with butter, brown bread Rice pudding, Pear	Poo normal Heat rash on neck 5.20pm
6.30pm	Breast milk	Rash gone

What are the basics I should record in the diary?

Time food is eaten	e.g. 1pm
Type of food eaten	e.g. banana or bread with butter
Type, length and severity of reactions	e.g. red rash on tummy 4pm, gone by 6pm
Medication given	e.g. 5ml Piriton, 4.05pm

You may also wish to include information about your child's general health:

- Degree of eczema, asthma, rashes, diarrhoea, constipation, colic etc. Are the symptoms better or worse today? Grade severity, e.g. 1-5 with 1 being mild and 5 being very severe.
- Other things your child has come into contact with that might cause a reaction – plants, animals, chemicals, etc.
- Sleep times and lengths, especially if the allergy is affecting your child's sleep.
- Crying when there is no obvious cause.

While I was introducing a new food every three days or so, I had a system of marking each entry with a big 1, 2, 3 or 4. That way I could keep track of which day I was on for each food because it could get pretty confusing. Once I knew a food was safe, I'd add it to my list at the back of the book for quick reference on those days when my mind was a blank! Alice

Tips for making it easier:

- Keep the diary to hand with a pen attached, in the kitchen or on the dining table for example.
- Fill it out while you and your child are eating.
- Take a mini-notebook if you're going out so you don't have to lug the big one with you. Keep it in your baby's change bag or in your handbag.
- Stick in ingredients labels from jars and packets that you use, for quick reference.
- Keep a list on the fridge or at the back of the diary of the foods that are safe.

Keeping a long-term food diary

If your baby has had a severe allergic reaction you may find yourself having to keep a food diary until you have finished weaning. Laborious as this is, when your child breaks out in hives or starts wheezing, having all those notes helps you quickly work out the cause.

You will quickly develop your own shorthand and become discerning about what is worth noting on a daily basis and what is just 'normal'. The diary is for you to use and interpret so do it *your* way, especially as it's going to be a big feature of your daily life. It can be as simple or as complicated as you choose. Understanding that its purpose is to help you pinpoint the foods that disagree with your baby will help you decide how much information to include.

Having to write down every mouthful you both eat can be a constant reminder that you have lost the natural, uncomplicated relationship with food you once enjoyed. However, as your fears settle and cooking and thinking about food in this new way becomes second nature, some of that old easiness will return. It doesn't take as long as you might think to start enjoying food again. Watching your baby enjoying new tastes and discovering what a mess he or she can make with food will be a great boost.

Childcare and food diaries

Ask your childminder or nursery staff to keep the food diary for you. This will undoubtedly require a more formal approach than your usual scribbling it in with a wax crayon!

- Drop the diary off with your child's food (and remember to collect it).
- Use a hardback book that can withstand being lugged about.
- Mark and label columns clearly.
- Check over the contents before you leave and ask the carer to explain anything you can't read or don't understand.

8 Shopping

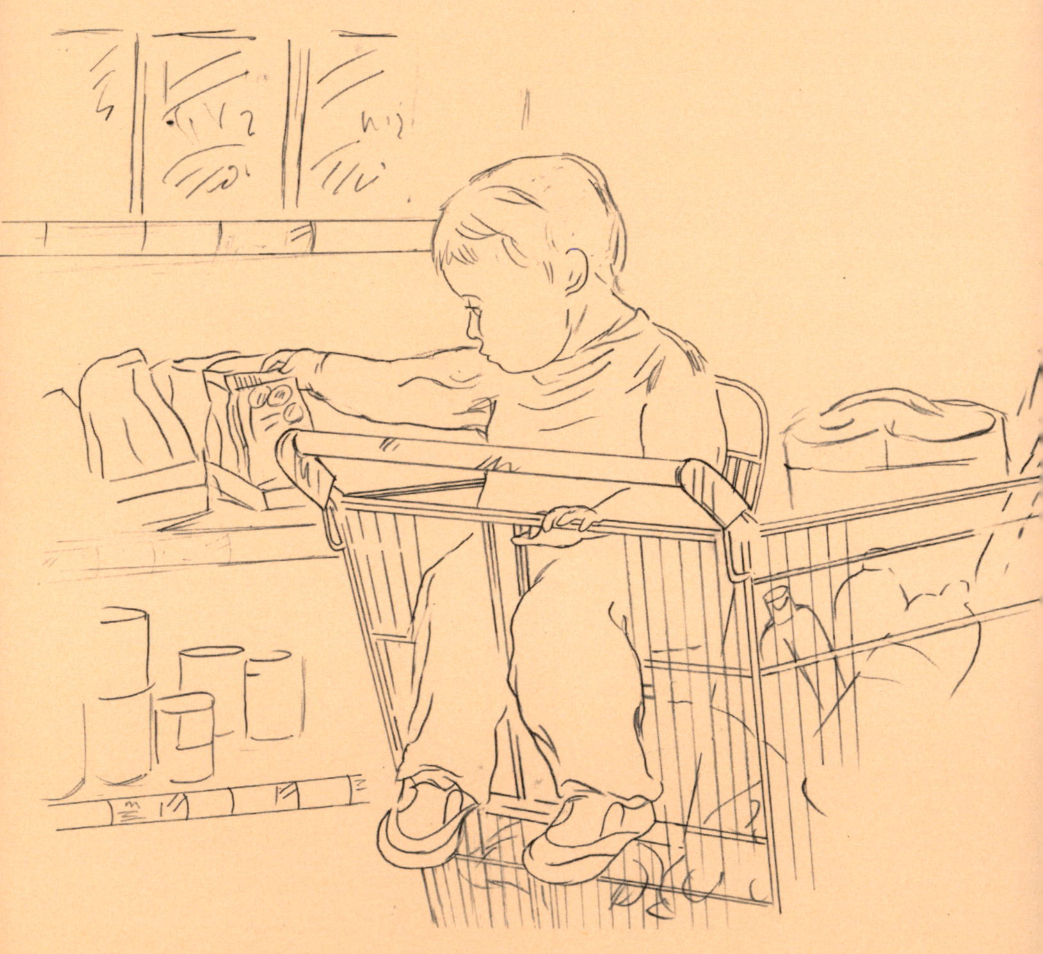

You aren't alone if you feel as though your child's life is quite literally in your hands as you stand in the food aisles. Don't despair: you will quickly learn to shop with confidence. The trick is to cut the task into manageable chunks and not try to tackle it all at once.

Learning to shop again

The quickest and easiest foods to shop for are those which have no added ingredients such as fresh fruits and vegetables, unadulterated cuts of meat or fish, milk, cheese, butter, eggs and flour. If your child can eat them, you buy them; if not, you avoid them. If only it were all so simple! The average shopping trolley contains a multitude of *apparently* safe, everyday items such as bread, yoghurt, packaged ham, pasta or margarine which in fact have to be scrupulously vetted.

Take plenty of time to check the ingredients labels. If you're not confident that you can remember all the different words that a food can be called, carry a list in your purse so you can double-check before buying. Dawn

Pretty soon, you will have learnt which types of food to pay special attention to and which you can count on to be free of your child's allergens. This speeds things up. If you buy mainly unprocessed foods you'll whizz round. However, if you tend to buy a lot of convenience foods then label reading – and therefore your shopping – will take longer. Avoiding allergens is often just a matter of buying the right brand. Once you've found the brands that are safe, it will get quicker, but remember to check the ingredients regularly as manufacturers do change their products.

Shopping with small children is nobody's idea of fun at the best of times. If you are also analysing each and every product that goes into your basket the job becomes more time consuming and considerably more stressful. For the first one or two shops after diagnosis, if you can possibly find somebody to mind your small children, you will find it much easier. If the thought of leaving your allergic child with someone else is too stressful, consider going shopping in the evening when your child is asleep or at the weekend, if you can leave him or her with your partner or another trusted family member.

Three-step programme to mastering shopping lists:

- Step 1: go to the supermarket *on your own* and pick up all the things you would normally buy. Make a note of all those that are still safe. Give yourself plenty of time.
- Step 2: request a supermarket 'Free from...' list and find safe alternatives for all the things you couldn't buy earlier.
- Step 3: put this information together to make your master shopping list, including a list of all the names your child's allergen can appear under.

'Free From…' Lists

Supermarkets and food manufacturers produce 'Free from…' lists to help people buy products which are free from major allergens including nuts, milk, eggs, soya, wheat and gluten. Ring the supermarket's Customer Service for lists (Appendix).

The whole list is too bulky to carry round as you shop because it includes every single safe product from fruit juice to frozen vegetables to bottles of wine. We suggest that you go through the list at home with a highlighter, select items similar to those you would normally buy and make your own list from that. Also, ask for up-to-date copies regularly as supermarkets do change their product ingredients from time to time. Some supermarkets will automatically send updates to their allergy customers, so ask yours if this is possible.

The lists are not foolproof and checking labels is still important but they do help narrow down the selection to products which ought to be safe.

Sadly, it is still the case that if your child has multiple allergies you will have to piece together a master list from all the separate 'Free from…' lists. Supermarkets do not provide multiple allergy lists.

I can't understand how in this day and age, supermarkets are unable to compile 'Free-from…' lists for more than one allergen. All the information is held on computer, sifting data is what computers do best. Why did I have to sit at home with my biro working it all out manually? It seemed so unnecessarily thoughtless, it made me cross. Alice

Bakery and delicatessen risks

Cross-contamination is far more likely to occur in a bakery or on the delicatessen counter because the foods which are safe are handled and placed alongside foods that are not. As a result, these present far more danger than packaged foods, and for severely allergic children the risk of buying these loose goods is too high. If cross-contamination is not an issue for your family, the 'Free from…' lists will tell you which foods should be safe. Also, as these foods are classified as loose, they do not have to keep to the new labelling laws. The safest option is not to buy items from bakeries and delicatessens (not even their packaged products) if you can buy the same item in a packet with an ingredients list.

Frustrations

You will be frustrated by the tiny print on ingredients labels, which can be obscured by packaging folds. You will be flummoxed by what goes into a simple cake. You will be annoyed by spillages on counters, the floor and the till belt. In short, your whole expectation of supermarket *convenience* may be challenged!

In the beginning shopping was a rollercoaster of delight or devastation – sometimes being thrilled that a product I wanted was safe or, on the downside, finding that I couldn't find an acceptable alternative for something. Shopping became a very long, laborious job reading the packet label on everything! Dawn

The thing I find most exasperating is sticky trolleys so that when Zac sits in the seat he's putting his hands in who knows what. These days I have my fruit and vegetables delivered and order all the bulky, storage cupboard stuff on-line. Sorted! Alice

I don't think it's good or practical for everybody in the family to avoid Thomas' allergens which means that I have to be extremely careful when shopping. I save a small section of the trolley for things which might spill and spoil the foods for Thomas. That way any chance of contamination from spilled milk, yoghurt or eggs is much reduced. Deborah

The 'Contains' or 'Allergy Information' labels on packaging are making shopping easier but even when you're an experienced label-reader, it's easy to make mistakes. Gwyneth accidentally gave her dairy-allergic son biscuits containing peanuts, which they had been advised to avoid:

I bought him some dairy-free Choc Nut Biscuits. On the front it said 'dairy-free, lactose-free, egg-free' so I picked it up. I didn't read the ingredients properly and of course it had peanuts in. I read it afterwards and thought, 'Help!' Luckily nothing happened. Gwyneth

The 'May Contain…' debate

How many people despair at this label? It used to be unique to nuts but is beginning to be used for other allergens, notably sesame, milk and egg. Of all the efforts the food industry is making on behalf of allergy suffers, this has to be the most unhelpful and contentious.

It is unhelpful, because customers want to know for sure whether a product does or does not contain a certain allergen, not that it *might*. It may be that the product is prepared or packed on a belt that also prepares a nut product or just manufactured in the same factory.

It is also contentious because in our culture of litigation there are those who are tempted to believe that manufacturers are just covering themselves against being sued. Whether this is true or not, the fact remains that unless manufacturing practices change, a small but significant risk exists which should not be ignored.

People who take the 'safe' option and avoid 'May contain....' labels often feel they are missing out on products which might well be safe for them if only they had a little more information to go on. For example, if you are allergic to raw egg but can tolerate cooked egg, a warning that the product 'may contain egg' isn't enough information. Likewise, if you are only allergic to peanuts but can tolerate hazelnuts, it is of no help to be told that a product 'may contain nuts' – what kind of nuts? Manufacturers are catching up, though, and are now trying to be more specific with warnings. Some companies are spending thousands of pounds creating entirely nut-free processing plants and should be highly commended for their understanding of the situation.

If you would like to support those lobbying for change in this area, join the Anaphylaxis Campaign or make a donation to Allergy UK. The more money they raise, the more campaigning they can do on our behalf. You can also write to manufacturers direct to voice your concerns – their addresses are usually printed on the packet.

Compulsory labelling of content

Manufacturers are required by EU law to label 14 allergenic ingredients[11] in a product no matter how small a component. This is a great improvement on the much hated 25% rule which preceded it, where allergens could be concealed in a compound ingredient if it only made up a small part of the recipe. It applies only to packaged food, so freshly prepared foods and loose foods from bakeries, delicatessens and catering establishments (such as restaurants, takeaways and hotels) are not covered. So whilst this content legislation is useful, there are downsides.

Professor John O. Warner says, 'Even if the likelihood that the constituent will cause an allergic reaction is vanishingly small, it must be declared. This, for instance, may well be the case for the use of highly purified peanut oil. Despite the fact that this will not cause an allergic reaction in peanut sufferers, the manufacturer will still be required to say that the product contains peanuts.' For those on restricted diets, this approach narrows the list even further. It seems allergy sufferers can't win when it comes to processed foods but overall this is solid progress.

Confused?

Some ingredients seem unsafe, but are they? Here we look at the most common questions.

Is coconut a nut? No. It is the seed from the coco palm.
Is nutmeg a nut? No. Nutmeg is also a seed and not related to the nut family.
How about water chestnuts? No. These are not nuts either.

The following ingredients do not contain milk protein and need not be avoided by people allergic to milk:

Calcium lactate	Cocoa butter
Calcium stearoyl lactylate	Cream of Tartar
Sodium lactate	Lactic acid
Sodium stearoyl lactylate	Oleoresin

Should someone allergic to egg avoid lecithin or E322? With the new EU labelling laws food manufacturers now have to state whether the lecithin is made from eggs or soya. When lecithin or E322 is used in food products it is usually derived from soya. Although it can be derived from egg, the quantity of egg protein present is not thought to be enough to cause a reaction even in the most sensitive individuals.[12] Egg lecithin is more commonly found in pharmaceutical products, so check with the pharmacist.

We avoided lecithin emulsifier and E322 for several years due to advice that they could contain egg. It was only when Professor Warner, at Southampton General Hospital, told us that they do not cause a reaction, that we were able to offer a much more varied diet to Lorie. Obtain as much information on which foods and additives contain ingredients your child is allergic to. Lilly

Should someone allergic to soya avoid lecithin or E322? Yes. The risk of a severe reaction to the allergenic proteins of soya in lecithin is small but real because it is made from *unrefined* soya oil.

Who should avoid hydrolysed vegetable protein (HVP)? HVP is derived most commonly from soya or wheat and should therefore be avoided by anyone with these allergies. Very occasionally HVP is derived from peanuts. The source of the HVP now has to be stated if it is one of the 14 allergens covered by the new EU labelling laws. Peanut allergy sufferers are advised to check the source of HVP before eating any foods containing this product.

Shopping summary

- Give yourself plenty of time – don't shop in a hurry.
- Buy fresh, unprocessed products for your family's meals.
- Make a list of the foods you know are safe.
- Try writing basic, weekly menus of dishes you can make easily and shopping lists to accompany them. Keep them and make a collection to use again.
- Look out for the useful 'Contains' or 'Allergy Information' labels on packaging.
- Keep any allergenic foods in a separate part of the trolley to avoid spills.
- Always read ingredients labels – ingredients can change.

9 Cooking and preparing food

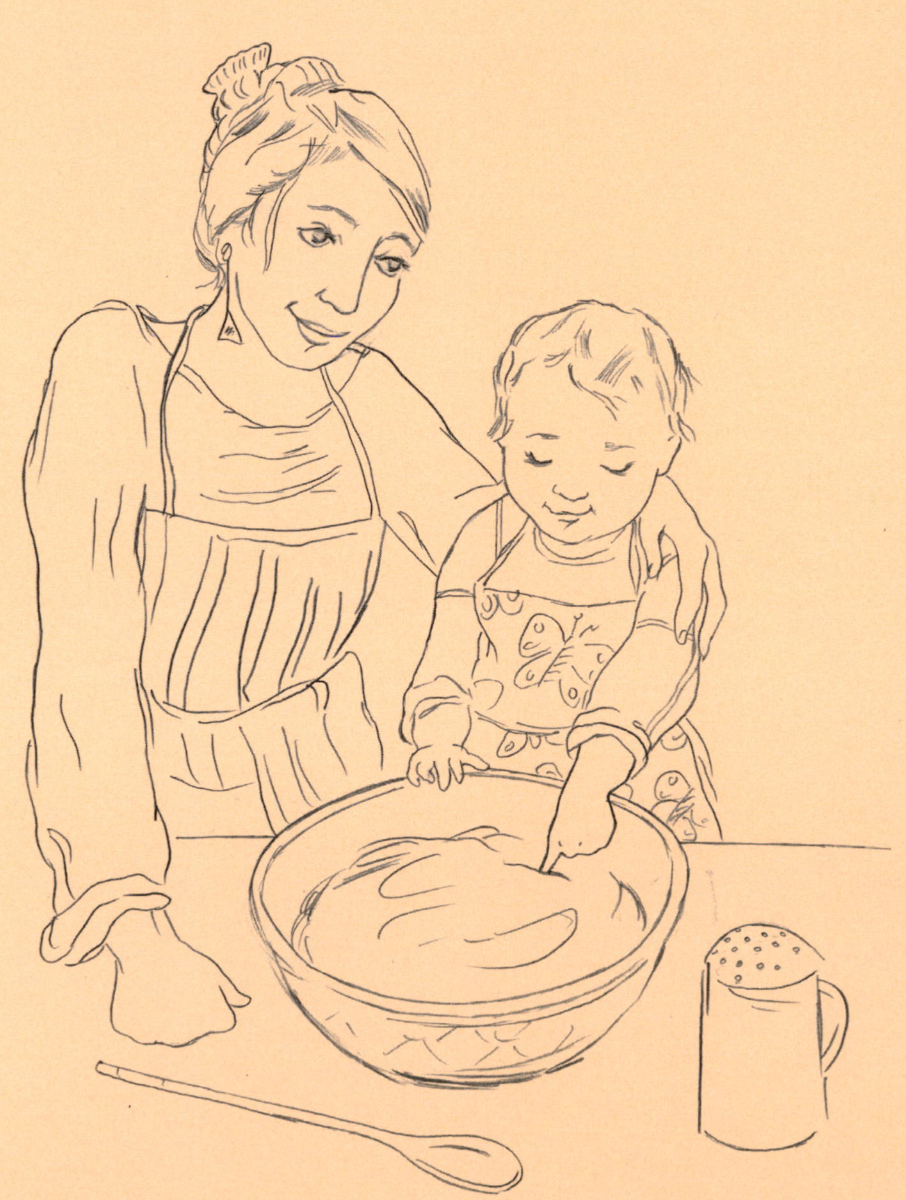

Should you cook separately for your allergic child or adjust all family meals to be safe? While they are very young, it is straightforward enough to make one meal for an allergic child and something different for yourselves. As your child gets older they will probably want to try what everyone else is eating. Having to completely re-think what you cook can seem pretty daunting.

One strategy is to make a list of all the 'safe' dishes you already know how to cook and start with them, gradually expanding your repertoire. Another trick is to choose dishes that can be adapted easily: for example the brand of sausage or margarine you used previously may no longer be suitable but another brand might be. Before long, you'll have your own recipe book that suits the whole family.

Cooking was tricky in the beginning. I wasn't the most experienced cook so I had to learn how to make things and how to make safe alternatives. I began to read recipes from books and magazines, and later from websites that offered allergy recipes. The thing I found hardest was that often a recipe would be dairy-free but not egg-free, or egg-free but not dairy-free. Substituting egg is the hardest, dairy products has been the easiest, but cheese is impossible! Dawn

Remember that if you cook and freeze batches of family food, they make great freezer-to-table meals in 20 minutes – the allergic family's equivalent of convenience foods. Shop-bought convenience foods without milk, egg, wheat or nuts do exist but not in great variety.

Peter is very accepting of his limited diet. I always bake lots of cakes and sweet treats so he doesn't miss out. He likes continental chocolate too. Angela

Multiple allergies

It is difficult enough managing one food allergy but some of you will have children with a severe allergy to more than one food. The more foods you need to avoid, the more difficult shopping and cooking become. Although the basic approach remains the same, you will need to work harder to find foods your child can eat and maintain a balanced diet. If you are struggling with this, seek advice and support from a dietitian (p.24) who can help you come up with a meal plan that suits your circumstances and budget.

In the early days, there will be times when you wonder if there is anything at all you can give your child to eat and feeding can be a little fraught. Make use of the supermarket 'Free From...' lists (p.82) and where possible ask for practical help from family and friends.

I used to listen to other parents moaning about their child's nut allergy and think, 'Can't you be grateful? I'd give anything to only have to deal with that'. I did know it was childish but I felt I was under so much more stress than them, having to cope with milk and egg as well as the nut allergy, plus asthma and eczema. Sometimes it was just so hard. Deborah

You, more than anyone, need the maximum support and help while finding your feet. Dealing with multiple allergies isn't easy but however unlikely it seems now, you really will get used to which foods you can give your child and it will become as routine as it does for parents of children with only one allergen.

TOP TIP

Some parents find that devising a weekly menu works well, particularly those dealing with multiple allergies. Deciding that Monday will be jacket potatoes, cold meat and salad; Tuesday – spaghetti bolognaise; Wednesday – chicken casserole and rice; Thursday – sausages and mashed potato, etc. removes some of the stress from shopping and cooking.

The family kitchen

Could any room in the house be more dangerous for an allergic child than the kitchen? If you *have* managed to remove all risk in your kitchen, well done! The rest of us need to think about how to tackle the common dangers such as chopping boards, utensils, the fridge, washing up, spills and crumbs.

We separate any foods containing Lorie's allergens and make sure we wash up thoroughly, using individual utensils. Tom

You will soon find your own ways of dealing with cross-contamination (p.14) and other kitchen dangers but here are our suggestions:

- In the fridge, store anything 'unsafe' at the very bottom – then it can't drip or spill on to 'safe' food. Put a child-lock on the fridge while your children are young.
- Either use separate chopping boards or find a glass one that can be washed thoroughly in very hot soapy water or the dishwasher.
- If your work surface is tiled or ridged, watch out for pieces of food lodged in the cracks.
- Wash up your allergic child's cutlery and plates first while the water is absolutely clean or put them through the dishwasher. Hot soapy water will clean away allergens; just swooshing under hot running water will not.
- When making sandwiches prepare your allergic child's first while the chopping board is still clean.
- Collect a plentiful supply of plastic containers with lids to separate foods safely.
- Have a special treats tin for your allergic child.
- Either buy safe biscuits for all the family or keep two biscuit tins.
- Insist that anyone preparing a snack in the kitchen clears up *thoroughly* after themself.
- Let your allergic child off washing up duty – there has to be one bonus to being allergic!

- When the oven is overcrowded, make a high-sided foil 'dish' for the allergic child's portion which you can then safely place on the same baking tray as other food.
- Always cook allergy-free dishes on the top shelf to avoid cross-contamination by spills from above.
- Make sure any unsuitable food or drink left out is pushed to the back of the kitchen surface – it isn't long before toddlers can reach up there.
- Change the dishcloth daily or whenever it has been used to wipe allergenic spillages. Scrubbing brushes can be put through the dishwasher. Use separate scrubbing brushes for allergenic and non-allergenic foods.
- Teach everyone to wash their hands and face before wiping them on hand or tea towels because severely allergic children may react after contact with contaminated towels. Keep aprons and oven gloves out of reach for the same reason.
- Eat at the table. Sweep up after each meal, especially whilst your allergic child is an inquisitive baby or toddler.

Producing meals that suit your allergic child's diet as well as everyone else's taste buds will mean less slaving in the kitchen.

The importance of your child learning to recognise danger foods

Learning how to recognise danger foods in the safety of their own home is not only essential but also reassuring for your allergic child. As he or she gets older, being able to spot potentially dangerous foods themself will be essential. Empowering them with that knowledge at home is a great start to keeping them safe and helping them manage their allergy successfully.

We can just tell Daisy something's got peanuts in it and she knows. We remind her by saying, 'Do you remember when you had to go to the hospital and couldn't breathe?' Fortunately she's the sort of child who is not particularly adventurous with food. She wouldn't instantly want to try something new, she's cautious. I don't know whether that's because of how she is or whether she's picked up on the fact that I'm careful. She often asks what things are and doesn't yet have opportunities to just go and help herself. Alison

Cook with your children

If you don't already, cook with your children, especially your allergic child. Let him or her help in the kitchen. Allergic children, more than others, need to learn how to handle and cook foods safely. It also provides great talking time and a chance to really interest them in the food you eat. Negative association with food can easily creep in for allergy families. Cooking together is a great way to dispel these fears. Get messy and enjoy!

Feeding non-allergic siblings

As far as possible, allow your other children to eat a normal diet, difficult as this may seem at first. Allergic children do have to accept that there are certain foods they cannot eat and learning to deal with this at home is a good place to start. It is tempting to make the whole house into a safe zone for the allergic child but that will not prepare them for life outside the home. Equally, siblings should be getting essential staples such as milk and wheat and they will learn to be safety-conscious around their allergic brother or sister.

Your approach to cooking for your non-allergic children may well be influenced by whether they are the firstborn or not because eating patterns for the family will be established accordingly.

Peter's younger sister, Alice, basically eats the same as him – she has soya milk and plain chocolate for example – but I give her things like cheese or yoghurt (which he can't eat) when Peter is at school.
Angela

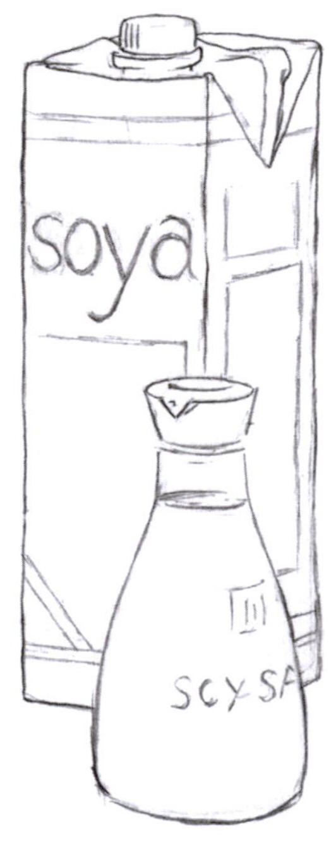

Non-essential foods such as ice cream, biscuits, cakes and chocolate can be bought or made allergy-friendly and shared by everyone in the family. However, don't make the mistake of always insisting siblings eat allergy-friendly foods because if they are forever denied their own choice, resentment can build up. It is also important that siblings encounter common allergens before eating outside the home, otherwise how will you know that they too are not allergic?

The exception to this is if your child has an allergy that is triggered by smell or the presence of an allergen nearby. For example, a reaction to fish that is triggered by the smell of fish cooking would be a very good reason to avoid fish in the house.

Like any other child, your allergic son or daughter will have likes and dislikes and is no less likely to have fads than the next child. There may well be good foods that your child can safely eat but if he or she does not like them, they will be off the menu too.

Food preferences

We all have likes and dislikes but many families also have particular food preferences for religious, ethical or cultural reasons. With the addition of allergy, these diets could easily become too restricted so seek the advice of a dietitian to ensure a balanced diet for your child.

Complacency

If, because of your fantastic care, your child does not suffer an allergic reaction for several months or years, you may relax and become a little too laid back. You might start to be sloppier with the chopping board, less scrupulous about items in the fridge or absent-minded about carrying adrenaline auto-injectors. This is an understandable reaction because deep down in all of us is the hope that our child will outgrow their allergy.

All we can say is that if your child has not been absolutely, positively, proven to have outgrown his or her allergy then vigilance must remain as high as ever. When we hear reports of somebody dying from an allergic reaction, it makes us all remember just how serious it is.

Certain that Thomas had gained a level of tolerance to milk, I slowly began to take less care with the risks of cross-contamination – until the day I put Thomas' dairy-free pasty one end of a baking tray and Isabel's ordinary chicken nuggets at the other end. During cooking, one of the nuggets slid down and touched Thomas' food but I dished it up anyway – surely that couldn't be a problem to him? 15 minutes later he had a swollen, blistered lip. How could I have been so stupid? It certainly taught me a huge lesson about never relaxing my guard. Deborah

As your child grows up

As your child becomes more independent he or she will need to learn to cope with the risks of allergy, understanding not only what he or she must not eat but also *why*, in order to tell other children and adults what could happen. If your child cannot remember ever having had an allergic reaction (no matter how severe it was at the time) he or she may not fully understand what all the fuss is about and be tempted to try the food in question to find out.

When I was eight years old, I hid behind the sofa and ate a tube of Smarties to find out what I was missing. I remember it very well because I was extremely sick for hours afterwards and weak for a couple of days. Amy (age 15)

I think allergy is really horrible. I really want it to go away. When I see other children eating things I can't have I want to eat some of it as well. I am tempted to try but I won't until I'm not allergic any more. I know I'd be very, very ill. I'd definitely have to go to hospital. Thomas (age 8)

It is common for children to underestimate the seriousness of an allergic reaction. As you try to explain it to them, you may find it hard to strike a balance between making them fearful and helping them to understand how ill they could be. Over time, with your help, your child will adapt and learn to live safely in their own way.

Finding alternatives and adapting recipes

To cook safely you need to know what can be substituted successfully and what can't. A lot of it comes down to trial and error which can be frustrating, so here are some tried and tested solutions other parents use.

Dairy products

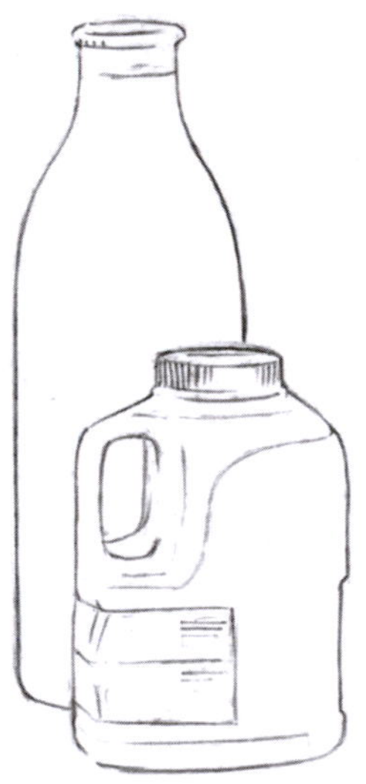

- Buy dairy-free margarine for cooking and spreading. It's not quite the same as butter but not bad. The Pure brand is good. Some normal baking margarines are milk-free and can be used successfully in baking.
- Soya milk makes great pancakes and Yorkshire puddings.
- Looking for an alternative to cheese? Don't bother!
- Soya cheeses can be used to add flavour to a soya white sauce for example. Some are designed to be eaten as 'cheese' and others to melt.
- Freeze olive oil in a little dish. It goes solid and is excellent to spread on bread.
- You can make a white sauce with soya milk although some people can tell the difference and say they don't like it.
- Soya white sauce works well for lasagne – you don't need the cheese.
- Use tomato-based sauces on pasta. Pesto is another good alternative if nuts are okay.
- In much baking and cooking, soya milk can be substituted for cow's milk.
- Swedish Glace is an excellent dairy-free ice cream available in most large supermarkets in a variety of flavours.
- Try chocolate flavoured ice cream sauces – many are dairy-free.
- You can buy dairy-free yoghurt in most supermarkets, usually made from soya beans. Buy the plain one and add fruit or try the flavoured ones. Some brands make junior versions with no bits.
- Dairy-free chocolate is too bitter for some children but they often like the minty ones. 'Ritter Sport Peppermint' is good, as are some brands of dinner mints but check the ingredients carefully, they often change.
- Plain chocolate chips are good for melting into shapes or adding to cakes.
- Make your own Christmas tree chocolates and Easter eggs by buying moulds. Find them online or in cookery shops.
- Kinnerton Confectionery produces a dairy and nut-free chocolate advent calendar which you can order from them in exchange for a donation to the Anaphylaxis Campaign.

Egg

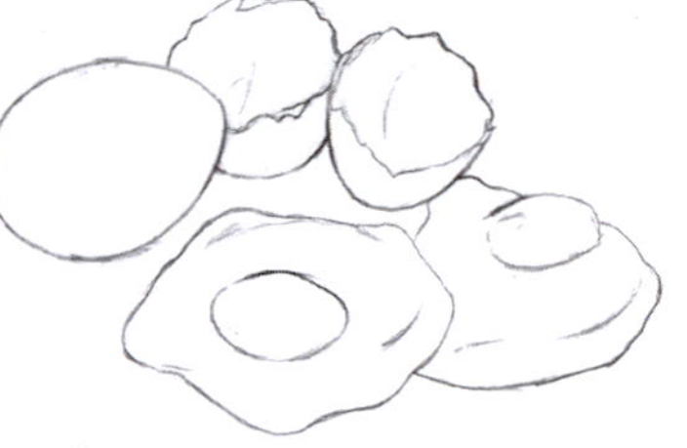

- Pancakes without eggs are fine. Add arrowroot powder or mascarpone for a lighter batter.
- Egg replacers don't live up to expectations and often produce flat sponges. Just make egg-free recipes instead.
- Chocolate Rice Krispie or cornflake cakes and flapjacks make great treats.
- In baking, eggs act as a binder and raising agent and also contain fat. One teaspoon of baking powder mixed with two tablespoons of water or milk and one tablespoon of oil is roughly the equivalent of one egg.
- There is no substitute for a boiled egg, an omelette or a meringue!
- Ordinary dried pasta rarely contains egg (check the packet) but the fresh stuff does.
- Instead of quiches make onion, fennel or spinach and feta cheese tarts. You can also make quite a passable quiche using tofu beaten into milk.
- Egg is added to some sauces and biscuits just to make them richer so you can often leave the egg out with no loss of flavour. Try adding in a little more butter or herbs or a splash of milk instead.
- Make custard with Bird's custard powder – good for trifles too.
- Blancmange is a good alternative to mousses.
- Use crème fraîche, cream cheese or yoghurt to make salad dressings where you'd usually use mayonnaise.
- Buy *Bakin' Without Eggs: Delicious Egg-Free Dessert Recipes from the Heart and Kitchen of a Food-Allergic Family* for all those cakes you thought you couldn't make any more but can. Brilliant! (Appendix)
- Visit the Allergy Buddies website for Alice's egg-free home-made recipes. (Appendix)

Wheat

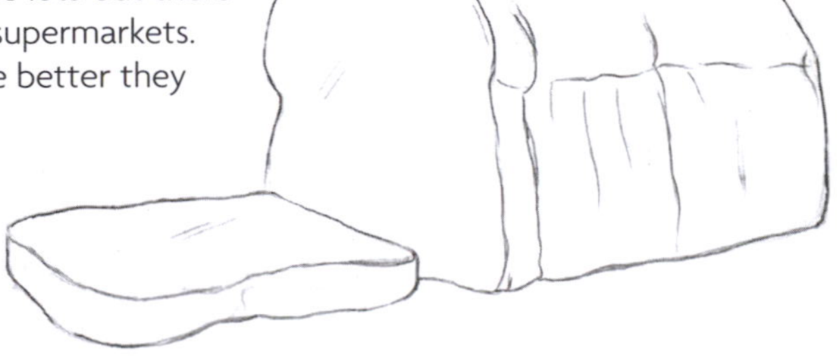

- Use gluten-free flours – there are lots out there and most are sold at the major supermarkets. Generally, the more you pay, the better they taste.
- Xanthum gum is an excellent addition to any baking because it provides the stickiness that is missing in gluten-free flours. Although quite expensive, it's more than worth it. It comes as a powder and you add a tablespoon or two. It really does get rid of the crumbling nature of gluten-free flours. It is available from www.goodnessdirect.co.uk and some health food shops.

- Polenta (corn/maize) makes an excellent substitute for wheat flour.
- Arrowroot is another wheat-free flour. It is good for biscuits and thickening too. Try Supercook's – their baking powder is also wheat-free.
- Cornflour is usually wheat-free but it is best to check as some manufacturers mix wheat flour in with it. Cornflour makes excellent shortbread.
- Chickpea flour, also called gram flour, is an Indian staple which makes excellent pancakes and onion bhajis. Buy it from Indian grocers or www.goodnessdirect.co.uk. It tastes a bit 'beanie', so mix it with cornflour or another wheat-free flour.
- Mix your own gluten-free flour with equal parts of potato flour, rice flour and cornflour.

Nuts

- Where cake recipes call for chopped almonds, use sunflower seeds instead.
- Ground sunflower seeds are good in biscuits and cakes too.
- Where savoury sauces call for ground nuts to thicken sauces, use a little cornflour instead.

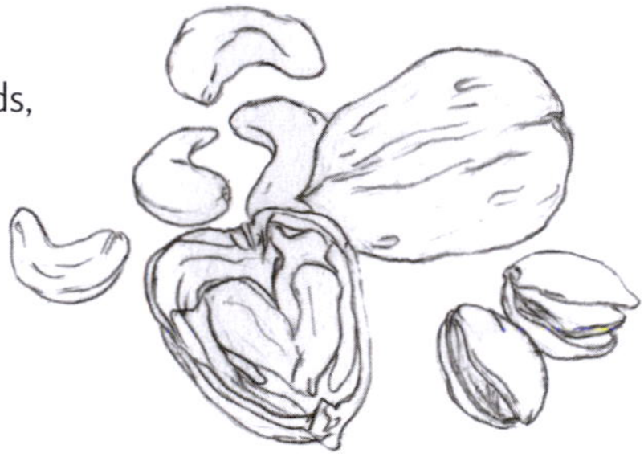

Weaning

Here are some alternatives to help make weaning with an allergy easier.

- Snacks and finger foods: soft dried fruit, soft fresh fruit, fresh veg, cubes of cooked chicken, bread sticks, rice cakes.
- Biscuits: bread sticks and rice cakes
- Spreads: jams, Apple 'n' Pear fruit spread, Marmite.
- Yoghurts for pudding: puréed fruits, shop-bought selections are good or make your own.
- Parboiled vegetable sticks: parboil vegetables sticks (carrot, parsnip etc) and freeze them. Grab a few before you go out, they'll be defrosted by the time you need them.

Final word

Before long, you will become quite an expert at feeding allergic children. You will still check ingredients lists but you will be much quicker at it. You will still try to find new and exciting foods or treats for your child but generally you will know what you can and can't buy. Shopping will become faster, (still slower than average but faster for you) and providing safe meals for the family will become second nature again.

Zac's story

by Alice

When people ask how I found out about Zac's allergy I usually reply, 'Well, he ate some egg and swelled up!' Zac was seven months old and was playing with a salad leaf with a dot of mayonnaise on the corner. A few minutes later his hands were bright red and the skin round his mouth was coming up red even though he hadn't eaten it. Quickly his hands, the area around his mouth, his cheeks and chin came up in small itchy hives.

We took him inside and rinsed the affected areas with cold water and agreed that this must be an allergic reaction to something. It didn't seem to be spreading and we were due to meet a friend, who is a nurse, so I thought I'd ask her opinion. She was more concerned than I had expected and stressed that allergic reactions usually get worse with each exposure. She said we should work out what he'd reacted to and be very careful. I remember naively thinking the worst that could happen was a bigger rash. We had no idea how serious it could be. I knew very little about anaphylaxis, not even the name.

We had given Zac egg a couple of weeks before, mashed hard boiled egg yolk, and he had had no adverse reaction although he hadn't liked it and had refused to eat it. I knew he hadn't had egg white (except the traces that must have been present round the yolk) so I rubbed a little mayonnaise on his hand and wiped it off immediately. Nothing happened, no rash, nothing. OK we thought, it can't be egg, must be something else.

Two days later, on Easter Sunday, we were at a family gathering for lunch and we had meringues for pudding (my favourite!). I gave Zac a tiny crumb of meringue. He thought it was yummy and of course wanted some more. I gave him another and then another to no obvious ill-effect so thought to myself, 'Oh well, he really is okay with the egg, he just didn't like the taste of it before.' My husband took Zac off to change his nappy. When they came back, Zac was bright red and rubbing his eyes ferociously.

We rushed outside where I could see him more clearly. He was crying and gasping so hard I couldn't tell if he was choking or just crying. His hands and face were bright red, covered in hives and swelling; within seconds his eyes were swollen shut and his face was a red, swollen mass, his features disappearing and his lips turning blue. He was very distressed. It was all happening so very, very fast. We really had no idea what we were witnessing and the only thing I knew about nut anaphylaxis was that constriction of the airways could cause collapse. I was assuming it was allergy because of what our friend the nurse had said earlier.

We didn't call an ambulance; someone rang the surgery which was, of course, closed on Easter Sunday. I remember being fixed on whether his mouth and throat were swelling too and on whether he could breathe. I had no idea he could be in serious danger from other symptoms of anaphylaxis. Reassured that he was breathing, we took him inside to bathe his face with a cold flannel to try to calm the redness down.

Zac was floppy and still horribly swollen but it didn't seem to be getting worse. After half an hour he began to calm down. I put him to the breast and, sobbing heavily, he fed a little bit which seemed to help soothe him. Gradually over the next hour the swelling came down and his features and eyes reappeared. He was still very red and puffy but clearly on the mend. We decided to take him home, over an hour away. He slept fitfully in the car.

When we came to get him out I noticed that his neck was the same angry red we'd seen earlier. Panicking, we stripped off his clothes and over the next hour-and-a-half watched as the hives spread over his whole body, everywhere they hadn't been a few hours earlier. He didn't swell up and he seemed much less bothered by the hives this time, rubbing where they itched but happy to play on our laps while we hurriedly consulted our baby books. Urticaria seemed to be the most likely diagnosis, which as far as we could work out just meant an itchy raised rash from an allergic reaction. We did what was recommended and put him in a cool bath with bicarbonate of soda to try and reduce the itching.

The more I read though, the more a niggling doubt kept coming back. The severe reaction my friend, the nurse, had talked about and the reference in the books to second phase reactions, breathing difficulties etc made us decide not to put him to bed without knowing what this was and what we could expect. We took him to the out of hours surgery where the GP diagnosed urticaria, prescribed an antihistamine – Piriton – and reassured us that he was unlikely to have any further reaction that night. He said we were to use the Piriton if it happened again and that many children had one unexplained bout of urticaria.

For the next three days Zac was hypersensitive to noise, easily startled, suddenly tearful for no apparent reason and not himself at all. When he managed to sleep he was jumpy, waking after 40 minutes in fright, crying, only to start the whole thing again. I breastfed him more than usual during the nights to comfort him and perhaps the egg in my breast milk aggravated his system further.

Seeing Zac acting so strangely for days afterwards bothered me; he clearly wasn't right yet. It also bothered me that the doctor saw Zac six hours after his reaction. The baby we presented to him did not look like the one who six hours earlier had seemed so seriously ill. It looked like a bad case of heat rash, nothing much to worry about.

Our local GP insisted that I had to find out what had caused the reaction but wouldn't refer me to a specialist for testing. He suggested that I go home, 'try a little bit of whatever I thought it might be' and watch for a reaction. After what had happened last time, did he think I was mad? I certainly thought he was and left the surgery angry and confused.

I had a child I didn't know for sure was allergic to egg, possibly other foods too, and no idea what I was doing. I began to wonder if I was overreacting, that perhaps the reaction hadn't been that bad after all. I got in touch with Allergy UK and they put me in touch with Deborah, another mother who'd been there too. Talking to her, I realised with a sinking dread that this was serious. We needed to see a specialist and quickly. We went private and off we went the following week, exhausted but hopeful that we'd get some answers and guidance.

Answers – yes. The skin-prick test showed that he was allergic to egg and he was prescribed adrenaline. Guidance – not much. We were told to only introduce new foods every three days, see a dietitian, keep a food diary, come back in three months and have him skin-prick tested again in a year. There would be a letter to follow. Three weeks later I was still chasing that letter. When it did finally arrive it was helpful, laying out the history of the allergy, the tests carried out and recommendations for the future - primarily to see a dietitian quickly and avoid a list of allergenic foods. But three weeks! That is 63 meals he had gambled his way through, not to mention the 63 meals that I had eaten, worried I might pass on an allergen through my breast milk.

Meanwhile, I'd been to my new GP, given him Zac's history and asked for a referral to a dietitian. He clearly couldn't see the point. 'Why? Egg is egg is egg. Just don't give him any egg!' I'd had enough of opinions, I wanted someone to tell me what to do. I came out feeling bruised and wobbly, definitely lacking the support I was looking for.

Zac's allergic reaction to egg undermined my confidence in myself as a capable mother. After all I was the one who'd given him the egg. Afterwards I felt really stupid. 'Fancy giving him that meringue' I heard my alter-ego saying, then 'but it was such a small amount'.

Without referral to a dietitian, I had to get on with working out how I was going to get Zac and myself onto safe, healthy diets. So began the painful and wearisome process of introducing a new food every three days, sequencing the food groups and keeping a careful record of everything we both ate and drank. We started with wheat, then dairy products, then meat. At a year old Zac was safely eating wheat, dairy products, meat and most fruit and vegetables. It seemed strange that only three months earlier I had been in a panic about him having an unbalanced diet and how it would affect his growth and development.

We stayed off peanuts and tree nuts until he was five and although he was allergic to nuts, he's okay now. He's had a couple of reactions over the years to things other than egg but nothing as serious as that first one. In all those years he's only had a tiny bit of egg white once by mistake, when he was five, and although he was very ill we didn't need to use the adrenaline that time.

As for the future, we remain vigilant about avoiding egg in all forms. We know he's seriously allergic to cats and we have learnt the hard way to avoid them or houses with cats. By the time he was three his eczema had gone. We have lovely, trusted friends who cook for him; friends' houses I know he can visit safely. He's been to stay on his own with his grandparents, gone for sleepovers with friends and he's been fine. We've been fine.

10 Socialising with an allergic child

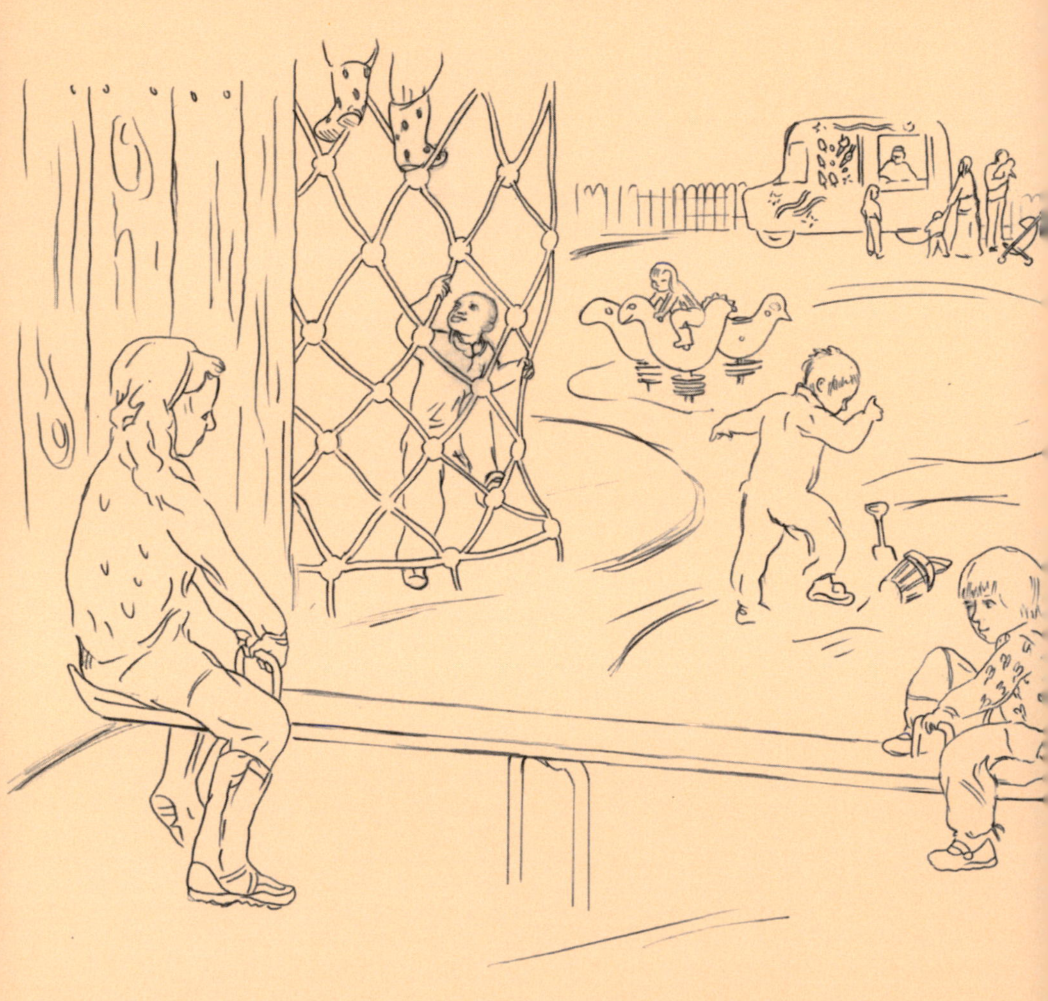

Once your child has been diagnosed with a food allergy, you quickly discover that it isn't only at meal and snack times that food allergy poses a problem. There are few environments that do not include food in one way or another – ice creams in the park; hot-dogs at the funfair; snacks on trains and buses; elevenses at playgroups and schools; food wrappers littering the streets. Cinema, theatre, seaside, you name it, there's food in abundance. This makes going anywhere harder work for allergic families but it is part of modern living, so unless you want to stay at home, it has to be faced.

In this section, we look at some common, social situations you will encounter, how to make the most of them and how to develop a confident allergy attitude in public.

Visiting family and friends

When you spend longer than a couple of hours visiting family or friends it is likely you will be offered food or a drink. Initially, the thought of somebody else catering for your child may put you off accepting invitations. We strongly recommend that you accept hospitality when it is offered because you will find that there is a great temptation to always host family and friends yourself simply because it seems to be the easiest solution all round. After all the hours you spend in the kitchen, imagine what a treat it will be to let someone else provide a *safe* meal. Here are some suggestions for making that possible:

- Provide friends and relatives you visit regularly with a safe shopping list for their local supermarket (p.82). Remind them to read the ingredients labels.
- Help devise menus that are safe before your visit. Some people will be relieved if you give them a selection of safe meals they can choose from. Others will have very fixed ideas about what they would like to serve and you can help them adjust these to be safe.
- Do take time to explain about cross-contamination (p.14) because this is an area people find hard to grasp.
- Ask your host to keep any packaging so you can check ingredients before the meal.
- Offer to take your child's own bread, margarine and milk where appropriate.
- As with travelling anywhere, take a supply of safe snacks in your bag.
- If your host seems to be struggling, check that you have explained about the allergy in detail. Remember when you didn't know where to begin? Encourage them to ring you with any questions, however small.

When you arrive, suggest that you run through the ingredients for the meal with the host well before it is served. This is reassuring for both of you. Even family and friends who have listened carefully to all you said and know what to avoid may make the occasional mistake.

Everything seemed fine, I'd checked labels and everything. As we sat down though, my mother-in-law said, 'I've put some nuts on the salad because it looked boring'. I was gob-smacked to say the least! Deborah

We don't have nuts in the house at all. My in-laws have peanuts in the house but they put them in a plastic pot with a lid on and it annoys me because I think you don't really need to have peanuts in the house, you can live without them. I mean, you don't have to get them out until Daisy's gone do you? But they think they're doing the best thing by putting them in a pot with a lid on. Alison

Keep it simple

If having your child's allergen around makes you nervous, ask that nobody eats it while you're there. One of the easiest answers is often a simple meal of potatoes, meat and vegetables with no fancy extras. Most allergic children can eat a roast providing there is no Yorkshire pudding (milk, egg and wheat) or stuffing (wheat, egg, nut or dairy products). Errors that might be made in cooking this meal for allergic children include:

- Butter on the vegetables – serve butter separately.
- Butter paper on the chicken – use olive oil.
- Ready-basted chicken or turkey (dairy products).
- Ready-stuffed joints (wheat, egg, nut or dairy products).
- Gravy granules (wheat, dairy products) – use cornflour to thicken gravy.
- Butter used to grease cooking dishes.

Alert your host to these potential problems in advance and run through them again when you arrive.

Puddings

Puddings are more difficult for other people to provide because so many include wheat, milk, eggs or nuts.

- Suggest a couple of puddings that are safe and supply the recipes.
- If your host is cooking pudding, remind them not to use butter to grease the dish (if dairy products are a problem).
- Suggest an allergen-free pudding that can be bought from their local supermarket.
- Offer to bring a pudding for everyone yourself or a single portion especially for your child. If only one part of the meal is different, your child will not mind – particularly if you take their favourite.

While I was still breastfeeding Zac and wasn't eating egg either (because he reacted to it in my breast milk) I used to ask my family to remove all eggy food from the menu for our visits and I made Zac batches of food in advance. That way we could all relax and enjoy each other's company at the table. Alice

Socialising with an allergic baby

As you start to socialise with your baby you realise how easily other people can forget about his or her allergy. Spotting potential dangers is unlikely to come naturally to them.

Even the closest of friends won't fully understand how you feel when you see your tiny, vulnerable baby next to something like a bottle of milk or a biscuit that could cause him such harm. You panic, your heart beats furiously and you want to declare the whole world unsafe for your baby. Deborah

The strain of keeping panic under check for the sake of a chat may make the idea of taking your baby out unappealing. The key to 'allergy socialising' is to start small. Ask your health visitor if she can suggest anyone with a baby of a similar age who might like to meet you.

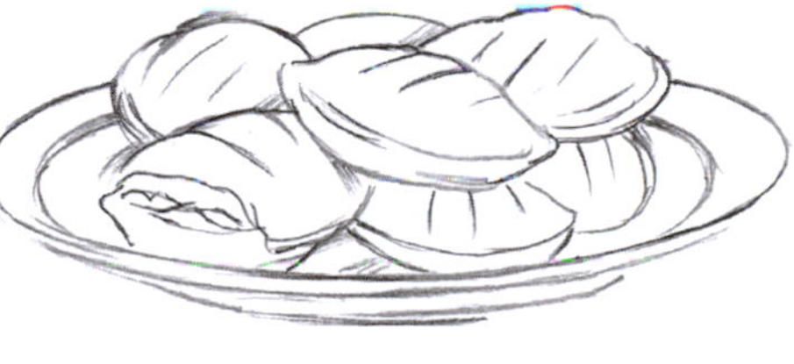

- Explore the established baby and toddler groups in your area as they are good places to meet new friends.
- Join a local Mother and Baby coffee morning group. You can host so that you have the chance to socialise in your own home which feels safe.
- If you find that you have a neighbour with a young child, say hello and ask her to come round for a coffee and chat. Many new mothers would love the opportunity to get to know another mum but lack the confidence to initiate a conversation.

Get-togethers where there are only babies of roughly the same age, like post-natal groups, are ideal because there will be no older toddlers dashing about to keep tabs on. However, most social gatherings for mums and children include children up to school age so learning to negotiate these will be useful. If you already have older children this won't be so daunting; for the first-time mother it can be a bit of a culture shock!

Matthew does ask if he can have this or that when we're out of the house or at playgroup. I say 'no' because it's got dairy products or egg in it. He just says, 'Okay'. Then his little brother grabs a bit and that's hard! Gwyneth

Mother and Baby coffee mornings in private homes

Smaller groups which meet in private homes are usually easier to negotiate than larger groups in a hall. One advantage is that you can ring the host in advance and explain your baby's allergy. You might discuss whether they would consider:

- Providing only raisins or fruit for the older children to eat.
- Helping you alert other mothers present to the allergy so they don't leave food or bottles of milk within reach of your baby.

Another advantage is that the opportunity to invite the group to your house will mean that at least sometimes, you can socialise in your own home where you feel safe. Ask people not to bring food – now is your chance to demonstrate that allergy-friendly entertaining is not only possible but just as much fun.

Being direct with people you barely know can be hard. If you want to attend coffee mornings in an effort to get to know other new mums you might feel awkward and worry about being difficult.

While I was breastfeeding, I was dairy-free as well so when I went to coffee mornings at friends' houses I'd be saying, 'I can't eat that, can't eat this, oh black tea for me' and I'd feel like I was making such a fuss. I felt self-conscious about it. It's sometimes difficult to make a fuss, especially if you're in someone's house where there really is nothing you can eat. Gwyneth

When I say she's allergic to this, this and this it sounds like I'm a totally neurotic mother. I can see people thinking, 'What else could she think of that she's allergic to?' Alison

TOP TIP

Being up-front about your child's allergy will make socialising easier all round. The first meeting is always the hardest but pretty soon friends and new acquaintances will be taking it all in their stride.

A special note on drinking cups and anaphylactic children

All young children will drink from any cup within reach which is particularly dangerous for your child. Keep your child's own cup out of the reach of other children and make sure he or she doesn't pick up cups or bottles belonging to others.

It's amazing how careless people can be with their children's drinks and food. I hated it even when I was only worried about my carpet but to be on tenterhooks because of my son's allergy was in another league altogether. Deborah

Toddler groups and playgroups

These groups are often stressful because of coffee time when biscuits, cakes and drinks are consumed. Baby and toddler groups held in large halls with little or no structure are the worst. With all those crumbs, dripping bottles of milk and sticky little fingers spreading food on toys, how safe you feel at a playgroup will probably depend on the severity of your child's allergy.

What makes for a good, allergy-friendly group?

- Staff who listen to your worries and are willing to make special arrangements to deal with your child's allergy.
- Sit-down time for snacks and drinks.
- Staff or mothers who walk round keeping an eye on what's going on and clear up spills and crumbs promptly.
- One where mothers are encouraged to keep a close eye on their children whilst socialising.

What should you watch out for?

- Children (or adults) helping themselves to cake and milk throughout the session.
- Food and spills on toys, the floor or chairs.
- Staff who do not understand the seriousness of your child's condition or can't make changes that would make the environment safe.

I visited lots of local toddler groups until I found one where the children were actively encouraged to sit down whilst they ate their snack and drank their juice. I also looked at whether the hall was clean, whether the toys were clean (no old biscuits lurking in boxes of toys or food smeared all over them) and at the general atmosphere amongst the mothers and the children. Once I found one I liked, I approached the organiser and explained our situation and offered to supply the toddler group with all the biscuits that they needed and that is what I do.

Dawn

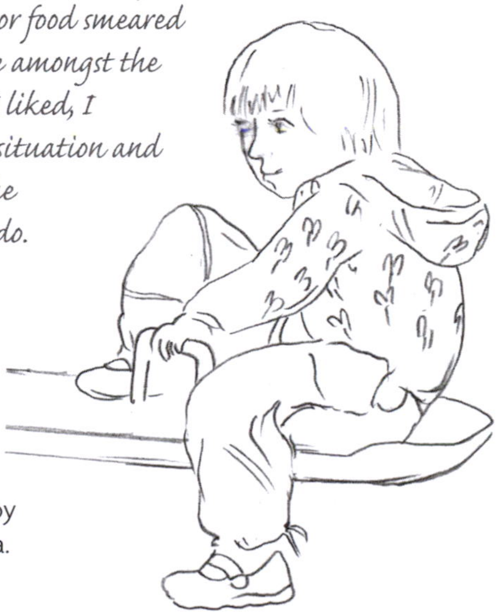

Avoid places that make you uncomfortable and never feel obliged to go anywhere just because you are expected to. What you can cope with will change over time, so every now and then review what you feel ready to do now. A group that felt unsafe for a crawling baby may work well for a pre-schooler and vice versa.

Playgrounds, theme parks and the seaside

Until you are responsible for a child with food allergies, spilt food or sticky equipment in public places are just an annoying inconvenience. For an allergic child however, these inconveniences loom large as sources of danger. It can feel as though letting your child play anywhere is going to be too difficult. You do need to watch out but try to retain some perspective. Play and fresh air are vital for children.

Tips from other parents:

- Carry baby wipes or a damp cloth with you to wipe sticky equipment.
- Seek out less heavily used play areas on busy weekends and bank holidays so it is easier to keep an eye on spilt food.
- Use beaches that are washed with each high tide. Occasionally food will have sunk or melted into the sand where it is not visible and endanger a severely allergic child. Going to tidal beaches where the sand is washed clean twice a day will reduce these risks.

Learning to face dangers calmly

When you are faced with unexpected dangers, try to contain your panic so that your allergic child will learn by example how to be practical about alarming food issues. This will allow your child as natural an upbringing as possible. Before you know it, your child will be alerting you to potential dangers!

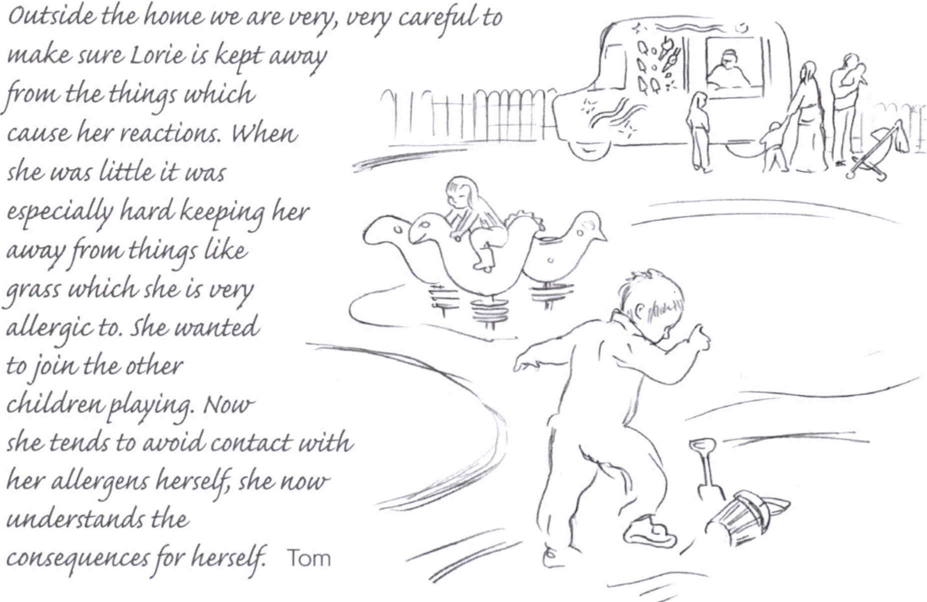

Outside the home we are very, very careful to make sure Lorie is kept away from the things which cause her reactions. When she was little it was especially hard keeping her away from things like grass which she is very allergic to. She wanted to join the other children playing. Now she tends to avoid contact with her allergens herself, she now understands the consequences for herself. Tom

Farms and zoos

When you are already busy thinking about medical kits, lunches, snacks and emergency procedures for a day trip, it's easy to forget some of the points below:

- Parents of children who are allergic to nuts or seeds need to check the feed in the little bags that are often available for children to feed the animals with. Elephant and pig feed is usually a selection of all sorts of scraps.
- Milk-allergic children should not bottle-feed calves, lambs or kids.
- Milk-allergic children should be kept well back during milking demonstrations.
- Egg-allergic children should not collect eggs.
- It is especially important for allergic children to wash their hands thoroughly after feeding animals.

Pet Food

While we are talking about animal food it is worth mentioning animals at home. Most young children like to help you to feed family pets and clean out their cages or hutches. It will be important to find out if any allergens are present in the pet food you use. Nuts and seeds crop up most commonly, particularly in hamster food. Cat food and fish food often contain fish. This is when those supermarket 'Free from...' lists that contain every product truly come into their own.

Bird feed usually includes seeds and nuts so if you want to continue feeding birds in your garden, give crumbs and currants instead. In other people's gardens, watch out for fallen peanuts on the ground under bird-tables or bird-feeders that little ones might pick up.

Lunch on days out

Thinking about where to have meals will be part of your planning for any day out. Picnics are a good option (p.111) but can be difficult in the middle of winter! Taking along food suitable for your allergic child to eat at a café or restaurant in case there is nothing suitable is another fall back. Many child-centred places sell lunch boxes, so depending on your child's allergies, these pick and mix options may work out well too.

11 Eating out and family gatherings

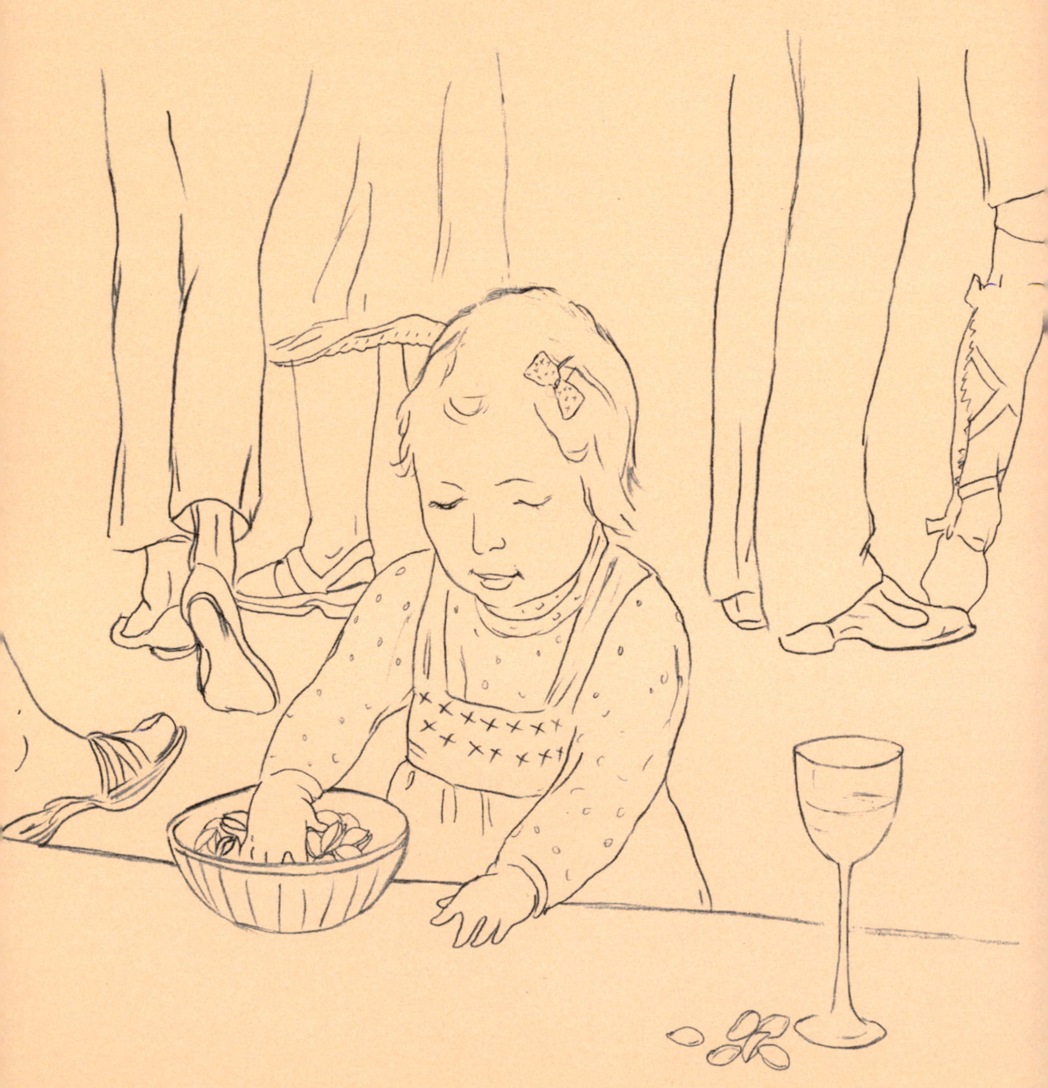

Although at first the prospect of eating out with your allergic child may seem impossible, don't despair. Even children with multiple allergies can be catered for.

The severity of your child's allergy will play a significant part in your approach to eating out. You cannot fully escape the risk of contamination so for anaphylactic children this may mean that eating meals prepared in a restaurant kitchen is just too dangerous. In these cases, take along your own food for your child so they can join in safely.

We don't eat out in restaurants much but on the few occasions we have, things have been fine. When the restaurant meal has been planned ahead, we have rung in advance and explained about the children's allergies. They have been very happy for us to take a snack in and have prepared vegetables and chips for the children, taking care not to contaminate them. Of course there is always an air of uncertainty but we carry adrenaline auto-injectors and mobile phones and this has worked very well. Dawn

Most serious allergic reactions to food happen outside the home so if the guidelines below seem over the top, think again. There is still widespread ignorance about food allergy, even amongst catering staff. Thanks to the hard work of allergy organisations and media coverage, staff are usually familiar with peanut allergy but be prepared for bewilderment when you say that your child is allergic to milk, eggs, wheat, fish etc.

McDonalds, which produces detailed ingredient lists, is okay if you pick the food carefully. At other places, when she was little I took my own food. Later on, I would explain to the waiter very carefully before ordering, 'If there is even the slightest bit of egg in her meal you will be calling for an ambulance, so please check and double check with the chef there is no egg.' Then I would try to order things that ought to be okay and then ask them to check again to make sure. Eating out has been a bit of a nightmare for us. Tracy

Increasingly, restaurants have allergy-aware staff, who can answer questions on ingredients and who will always check finer points with the chef (for example whether the oil being used to fry your child's food has previously been used to fry nut or egg products). The responsibility will still be with you to flag up these problems and the guidelines on the following pages should equip you to ask the right questions.

We choose carefully from the menu, ask the waiter to check our choices with the chef to make sure there are no eggs or nuts in the food we've chosen for Zac. In many cases, staff have gone out of their way to help, once they understand how serious it is. I'm still surprised by the thoughtfulness of others. Alice

The golden rule is: absolutely *never* eat out without your child's adrenaline auto-injectors to hand.

Fast food

Fast food chains are frequently condemned for serving unhealthy food but can be a haven for allergic families because they provide the *same* meals with the *same* ingredients nationwide. Even better, most of them also produce a food ingredients list which you can pick up at the counter.

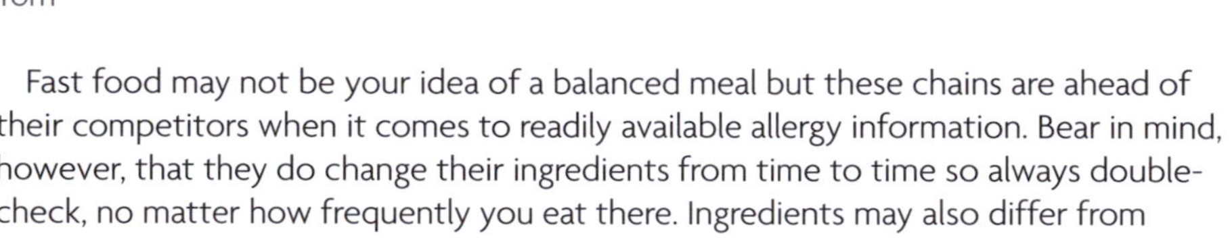

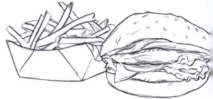

We were quite determined Lorie would be allowed to go to McDonalds with her friends. We contacted their head office and they were very helpful in listing the ingredients they use. Tom

Fast food may not be your idea of a balanced meal but these chains are ahead of their competitors when it comes to readily available allergy information. Bear in mind, however, that they do change their ingredients from time to time so always double-check, no matter how frequently you eat there. Ingredients may also differ from country to country.

Discovering that the batter in our fish and chip shop didn't contain egg was brilliant. I'd always assumed that batter of any sort contained egg but when I asked, they produced a packet of something called batter flour which they just mix up with water. Alice

Canteens and cafeterias

Canteens can be tricky because there always seems to be pressure from the mounting queue and serving staff to rush through as fast as possible. Staff don't always know what is in the dishes on offer and talking to them over the high, glass counters can be very difficult. It is always awkward having to discuss your child's allergy at the top of your voice, when there are people waiting impatiently behind you. So don't stress yourself out. Instead:

- Go at a quiet time, early or late lunch for example, so that you can ask for ingredients details without feeling under so much pressure.
- Choose foods that you know for certain cannot contain your child's allergen even if this means a very restricted meal like chips or a baked potato.
- Explain to the person serving that your child is allergic to some foods and you would be grateful if they could serve your food with fresh utensils to avoid cross-contamination.
- Particularly for multiple allergies, asking to read the ingredients labels yourself may help too.

I don't trust the staff to check the ingredients properly because of the different names milk comes under, like casein or whey, so I ask them to bring me the box or packet so that I can read it myself. Deborah

Cafés, bistros and restaurants

Cafés, bistros and restaurant chains are a popular option for families. Planning ahead makes eating out much easier, not only for you but also for the staff. You will have time to decide whether to find somewhere else if you doubt the restaurant can cater safely for your child.

- When booking a table, explain about your child's allergy and see how they react. Are you treated sympathetically? Great. Are you misunderstood? Steer clear!
- Children's menus often include pizza, chicken nuggets, fish fingers, hamburgers or sausages. The packaging the foods were supplied in will list the ingredients. You may wish to insist on reading them yourself, particularly for allergens that can appear under different names.
- If ingredients lists are not available, ask if the chef can recommend a dish that would be suitable or cook something special but be realistic and offer suggestions. Most people with multiple allergies can eat plain, grilled chicken or steak, with boiled, roasted or chipped potatoes and unadorned vegetables.
- The first member of staff you are likely to meet is the waiter or waitress. Don't expect them to understand about food allergy and the importance of avoiding any trace of your child's allergens. If you are unsure that they will explain your concerns to the kitchen staff properly, ask to speak to the chef directly.
- Make a small laminated card listing in alphabetical order the ingredients to avoid. You can then hand this to the waiter who can take it to the kitchen to check with the chef.
- For severely allergic children, make sure that the kitchen staff understand the risks of cross-contamination and are prepared to use separate cooking utensils and pans where necessary.
- Ask for any spills and crumbs on the table, chairs and surrounding floor to be cleaned up, and check that the cutlery is clean.
- High chairs are a particular risk because they never seem to be properly cleaned. Wipes are ideal for cleaning under, over, down the sides and in between the beads and twirls. Don't be worried that you'll upset anyone; little fingers get into every nook and cranny.

A friendly waiter tied a helium balloon to Zac's highchair which he tugged at happily and batted about. It wasn't until we got up to leave that I noticed the chocolate cake smeared on the top. Another lesson learnt. Alice

Ask kitchen staff to watch out for the following:

- Cross-contamination from grill pans, griddles, saucepans, utensils and chopping boards that have been used for other foods; oil previously used for frying food containing nut or egg; unsafe food dropped accidentally onto your child's dish.
- Hidden ingredients in pre-prepared sauces, marinades, puddings and bases.
- Garnishes that might include your child's allergen.
- Butter on vegetables or used to pan-fry food.
- Sauces, dressings or toppings that include your child's allergen.

A friend ended up using her Italian allergy translation cards in a restaurant in London when it turned out the chef didn't speak a word of English. They'd just come back from a holiday in Italy and she still had them in her bag. Alice

TOP TIP

One thing you learn quickly is that being over-protective is okay – in fact it is essential.

Unplanned meals out

There are occasions when you cannot book a table in advance or talk to the chef ahead of time. It can be awkward to walk out of a restaurant or café when you are all seated. The simplest solution is to go in ahead of the others and find out whether the restaurant is suitable. It is then easier to move on elsewhere if necessary.

When a meal has been more spur of the moment, we have looked for a clean restaurant and ordered only chips. We have had no bad experiences. Dawn

If you drop in, you will have to work harder at checking ingredients and bear in mind that if you arrive at the peak of the lunchtime or evening rush you cannot expect as much help and co-operation as at quieter times of the day.

Thank you

When you've had a good experience, it is always worth making a special point of thanking all the staff for their help and understanding. They'll be sure to remember you and other families like you.

Picnics

Love them or hate them, your children probably think picnics are great. Parents of allergic children need to become expert at packing picnics.

Whether you are enjoying a day at the seaside, in the countryside, at the park, in a theme park or at the zoo, the picnic is an essential part of the day not least because for allergic families it may well be the only reliably safe source of food available.

Where to picnic

Think about where you are going to have your picnic. Halfway up a remote mountain or on a deserted beach far from civilization is probably not the wisest choice but anywhere accessible should be fine if you have antihistamine, adrenaline and a mobile phone available. If you are going for a walk in remote countryside be prepared to give a grid reference from the map should you need to call an ambulance – it will help them to find you quickly.

What to eat

Picnics are not the time to try new foods. Take food that you know you can rely on, food that has been eaten by your allergic child many times before. If you are sharing a picnic with friends make sure your allergic child sticks to what you know is safe however tempting it is to try something that looks great and seems okay (unless you can check ingredients). Play it safe and enjoy the occasion.

Be particularly careful about cross-contamination. Plates are easily contaminated on a picnic where everybody is passing round and helping themselves to a variety of food.

Wasps and bees at picnics

The scourge of all picnics, wasps and bees can make outdoor eating in the summer months impossible for those allergic to their stings. A common fear among parents of atopic children is whether wasp or bee stings will cause a severe allergic reaction. Allergic reactions to insect stings can occur at the first exposure so this fear is not unfounded. The key tips for successfully sharing your picnic with wasps and bees are:

- Avoid fizzy drinks, beer and sticky buns.
- Place something sweet and sticky a short distance from the picnic to attract the wasps away from the food.
- Encourage your allergic child not to flap their arms. This will only anger the wasps and make them more likely to sting. The adults should try to remove the wasps whilst the allergic child remains still.
- Avoid eating outside in the heat of the day – breakfast and supper picnics are fun options.

See the Anaphylaxis Campaign website for more information; for a personal view see www.insectstings.co.uk.

Family gatherings

These events pose a particular problem because you may feel you can't say no, or don't want to miss out. Elsewhere we have looked in detail at helping other people to cook safely for your child (p.99) and food options for birthday parties (p.149), all of which apply here, so do read those sections to pick up other tips. Family gatherings do bring different challenges, which we look at next.

Self-catering

For special family gatherings, food will undoubtedly play a central part. Celebrations are a time to bring out traditional recipes and treat everyone to special dishes which usually include your child's allergens in abundance.

It will not always be appropriate or possible to adapt recipes to children's tastes or to be allergy-free. This means your child will miss out but lots of non-allergic children are fussy eaters and often refuse adult dishes, like Christmas pudding or strongly spiced dishes, so it's not unusual to see children either with a limited selection on their plate or an alternative. You could always suggest to the host that you bring a pudding or savoury dish that all the other children might like too, then your child won't feel like the odd one out.

If it is a 'bring and share' gathering it may not be feasible to organise for everyone to bring suitable food. Take your own provisions for your child and unless you are *sure* a dish is safe, just give them their special box.

Pre-dinner snacks, canapés and other nibbles are a huge worry. Not only are they always the last thing hosts consider, but guests drop bits on the floor and even on your passing child's head! Finger foods bring the added concern about guests touching your allergic child with allergens on their fingers, or worse passing them something that should be safe and contaminating it. Alice

These are the small details that we worry about but which wouldn't even occur to someone who hasn't lived with severe allergy. The best policy is to remember to mention the issue to your hosts and see if allergy-friendly versions are possible. As ever, offer to provide a selection yourself.

Caterers

Where the food is to be brought in by caterers, can you obtain the telephone number of the caterer to talk to them direct? They are usually well clued-up on different dietary needs and will be able to cook your child a suitable meal. Use the same guidelines as eating in a restaurant (p.109).

Buffets

Ask the hosts if your child can be first in the queue before the safe food has run out or been contaminated by serving spoons being moved from one dish to another.

Younger children need special attention

The worst time for socialising is the toddler years when children are on the move but not yet allergy aware. Going along to an event invariably means following your child around to ensure they are okay and not getting a moment to talk to anybody, let alone enjoy yourself. After making sure your child doesn't eat anything they shouldn't, the next biggest concern is accidental exposure.

Because Matthew's eczema was so obvious and people could see how bad he looked, it acted as a bit more of a trigger for them not to feed him anything. Gwyneth

If there is allergenic food around, you're constantly on the look out for other children walking around with food or washing off in the paddling pool; your toddler tripping into someone's plate left on a chair, eating crumbs off the floor or other people's discarded plates; even food being dropped on his or her head. All this means parties and gatherings can be very stressful and you can end up feeling flustered, hating the whole experience and wishing you could go home.

Life was hardest when Lorie was two or three years old and she would often cry because she didn't understand why she couldn't have the same things as everyone else. Tom

As each year goes by, your child will become more allergy aware and, with your help, more conscious of what the dangers are and how to avoid them – so will the rest of your family. Meanwhile, if things are so stressful that you are considering turning down an invitation, you could try:

- Planning beforehand to share the toddler – chasing with your partner, family or friends for a set period of time so that you have a chance to enjoy uninterrupted conversation and a bite to eat yourself.
- Asking a friend or family member to look after your allergic child for the day and going alone.
- Taking it in turns with your partner to attend social gatherings and then inviting close family to your house in the near future so that they don't miss out on time with their young, allergic relative.

I'm from a large family and we all get together regularly. I've always asked if food can be allergy-free and I have noticed that as the years have gone by less allergenic food appears at the table. This is partly because Zac is growing up and they naturally see that he wants to eat more of our food now but also because my family are just getting better at coping with his allergy. It certainly makes these occasions easier and less stressful for us, and for them I think. Martin

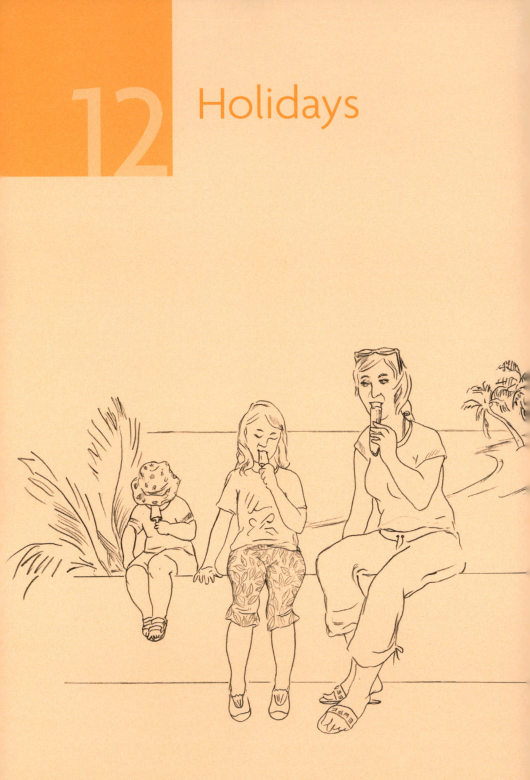

12 Holidays

A surprising number of the parents we interviewed haven't been on holiday since their allergic child was born. 'Why? Surely it can't be that difficult to arrange?' comes the cry from people who don't understand.

I would love to stay at a hotel with the children or go out for meals more often but it is hard work. Whilst we know that with lots of discussion between us and the chef we will eventually get served an appropriate meal it seems a lot easier to go self- catering when we're away from home. Angela

Concerns over leaving the safe environment of home, relying on hotel catering, shopping for groceries in a foreign country, coping with language barriers and the logistics of the journey itself can seem like a recipe for the *most* stressful two weeks of the year. It needn't be like that though. With a little forward planning, holidays are possible.

Holidaying in Britain

Self-catering

The easiest holiday option is self-catering. Meals need be no different from the food you would prepare at home, giving you peace of mind. The obvious drawback is that you will still be cooking every day and not getting the break that a catered holiday would provide. However, you can take holiday short-cuts like buying a ready-cooked chicken, pre-packed cooked meats and oven chips.

When we go on holiday, we go self-catering, usually to a caravan park. We always book a new caravan and go early in the season so we know that the caravan hasn't been used very much. When you have children with asthma and eczema the cleanliness of the upholstery and curtains is very, very important. We find out where the nearest Tesco is as that's the shop we know and are already familiar with the brands they stock. We also find out how far the nearest hospital is from where we are staying. Dawn

Find out in advance, via the local Tourist Office, which supermarket is closest to your accommodation and ring for that supermarket's 'Free from...' list. To make shopping easier, highlight the products you are likely to buy and compile your own list (p.82). You can book accommodation that is smoke and pet-free and take your own bedding if asthma and eczema are also a problem.

Hotels and guest houses

Staying in a hotel is perfectly possible with forward planning and good communication. Many hotels and guest houses will make sure that your child can safely eat the food provided once they know what you need.

- Telephone the establishment before booking and speak to the manager. Explain exactly what would be required should you stay at the hotel. If the conversation leaves you with concerns that they cannot address, try another hotel.
- Follow up the booking with a letter to the chef, and a copy to the manager, clearly stating which foods and ingredients must be avoided in order to keep your child safe. Give suggestions of alternative foodstuffs if you feel this will be helpful.
- Arrange to speak to the chef before confirming your booking to be sure that he or she understands all you said in your letter.
- When you check in, ask to see the manager and be introduced to the chef and remind him or her about your child's allergy. (See also p.109 on restaurants.)
- Many hotels will supply soya milk or store it for you on request. Check that the fridge is accessible in case you need milk during the night.
- When you check out make a point of saying thank you. The trouble they have taken will have made your holiday possible and paved the way for other allergic families coming after you.

Bed and Breakfasts

Ring in advance to discuss your child's allergy and what might be suitable from their breakfast menu. Alternatively, suggest bringing your own cereals and milk.

Take as much stuff with you as possible but check this is okay with the people who run the B&B. For example, a place may not be receptive to you taking your own food and if that's the case, take your business elsewhere. You will find somewhere that is fine. Most places are more understanding when it's a child. Dawn

Staying with family and friends

Although there will be more meals to consider, the advice in *Visiting family and friends* (p.99) is just as relevant whether you are staying for one meal or many.

If you have children who suffer from asthma and other allergies, for example to pets, feathers (pillows and bedding) and mould (windowsills, bathroom carpet), nobody will mind if you take along your child's own bedding but the other allergens are more difficult to avoid and often you don't know about them until you arrive. Make sure you have plenty of your child's medication available. Ask your doctor about giving a little extra asthma medication or antihistamine to your child whilst away if you feel it may be required. Don't be surprised to find that unfamiliar environments make your child more wheezy than usual. It's hard to predict beforehand how they will react. Take sensible precautions and try to strike a balance between limiting your child's exposure and having a normal life.

Holidaying abroad

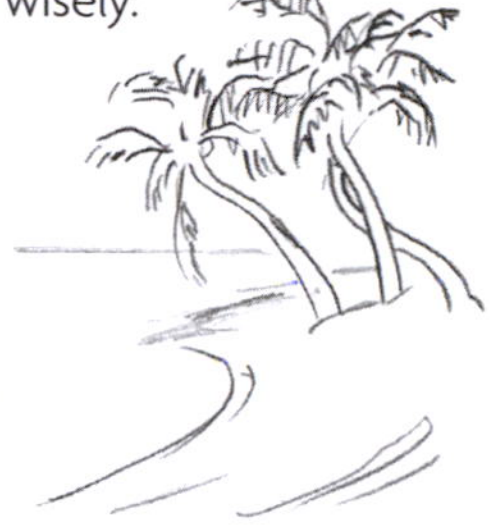

The key to holidaying abroad is to choose your destination wisely. Nut-allergy sufferers will find much of Asia a real challenge and trekking across Mongolia would not be the smartest choice with a milk-allergic child!

We went on holiday to Munich and I was dreading the catering aspect but actually this turned out fine. Angela

Self-catering

This is the safest option because you can prepare meals using similar ingredients to home. Beware kitchens that are too basic. If you are intending to cook most of your meals, you would be well advised to check with your travel agent that the kitchen includes a hob, oven and fridge. Apartments owned by neighbours and friends are a good option: they should be able to recommend local shops and restaurants and even a friendly neighbour to call on for help.

Packet foods often carry an English translation of ingredients, making them a convenient way to choose safe foods in foreign supermarkets. Also, look for local markets where the produce will be fresh and the producer can answer any questions you may have about different foods on the stall.

Hotels and restaurants

Self-service, buffet style catering cannot be guaranteed safe for allergic children as cross-contamination from serving utensils and food dropped onto other dishes is highly likely. Choosing a hotel with a waiter-service restaurant instead is preferable.

The precautions necessary for eating in restaurants abroad are the same as for restaurants at home (p.109), except that the language barrier may make clear communication difficult (see *Translation cards* p.118). If in doubt, keep your child's food simple: plain grilled meat with potatoes or rice and vegetables, for example. If your child has a milk allergy remember to check that vegetables and other foods are not tossed in butter.

We managed to eat out very successfully in Greek tavernas until one evening at the end of the holiday. I went through the usual routine of explaining the situation and the waiter very helpfully told me that the rice was cooked with butter. I asked for a jacket potato instead for Thomas' meal. When it came, the jacket potato was there alright but so was the rice! I asked for a new meal but I think they just scraped the rice off. Deborah

To a child, there is nothing wrong with repetitive, simple meals as long as they are his or her favourites.

Half-board in a hotel in Portugal was difficult. Matthew lived on chips really, plain pasta, things like that. Our single biggest difficulty was finding safe food. Gwyneth

Take loads of snacks, speak the language and don't worry too much about them having a balanced diet – they can survive on fruit and bread and chips for a week if needs be. Angela

Puddings
If your child cannot eat the puddings available then why not wait? Pay for your meal and then buy a pre-wrapped lolly or ice cream for the children on the way to a bar for a drink. Or walk along the beach or sit by the pool with a treat from the shop.

Translation cards

In countries where you don't speak the language, make use of Translation Cards available from Allergy UK. A set of three laminated cards is provided, each about the size of a business card. The cards contain an Allergy Alert message, an Emergency message and a message for use in restaurants to ensure that your food order is free from the particular allergen that causes your severe allergic reaction.[13] Similar cards are also available from YellowCross and Kidsaware.

I took a sheet of phrases with me like, 'Has this got milk in it?' and 'My child is milk-allergic'. I'd found a programme on the internet where you could type a phrase in and it would come back translated. Gwyneth

There are websites that offer this type of translation service for free but as the disclaimer will tell you, they do not offer a perfect translation and are not a substitute for a competent human translation. If you already speak the language Action Against Allergy has a table translating key words for the most common allergens into French, German, Spanish, Italian, Greek, Dutch and Portuguese.

TOP TIP

Find out the number used to call for an ambulance in the country you are visiting. Check with your network operator that your mobile phone will work abroad.

Taking your own food abroad

Check with your travel agent about any possible problems with customs if you intend to take your own food on holiday. If your child uses soya milk or other alternatives carry them as hand luggage so that they don't get lost but there are rules on what you can carry as hand luggage, so you will need to check hand luggage restrictions with the airline before departure.

When we went self-catering abroad we took a lot of food with us. Matthew could eat toddler meals in jars at that time so it was fine. Gwyneth

Medication

Make sure that you carry a plentiful supply of any medication your child might need. If you are worried that you will not be able to replace adrenaline auto-injectors whilst on holiday, ask your doctor for extras. If you keep adrenaline auto-injectors at nursery or school you can use these as extras (just remember to put them back on your return).

One of my concerns about travelling abroad with Zac is that we may not be able to find the medical care he would need if he had an anaphylactic reaction or that we might not understand well enough the treatment he'd be given. Having said that, I do remember that before Zac was born I used to worry about other travelling scenarios such as one of us becoming very ill, or the plane falling out of the sky. Strange how I never seem to worry about that sort of thing now! Alice

I did notice that I made a mental note of pharmacies wherever we went! Gwyneth

Travel insurance

Most standard policies do not insure for pre-existing medical conditions, including asthma and anaphylaxis, so you will need to find a policy that will cover your child's allergy.

The British Insurance Brokers Association will give you the names and telephone numbers of insurers who deal in specialised travel insurance but these tend to be quite expensive. For more economical insurance try the big insurance companies and *check the small print* with them before buying.

For European cover, take a free European Health Insurance Card (EHIC) with you. You can find out more about this and apply online (Appendix) or at a post office.

13 Travelling

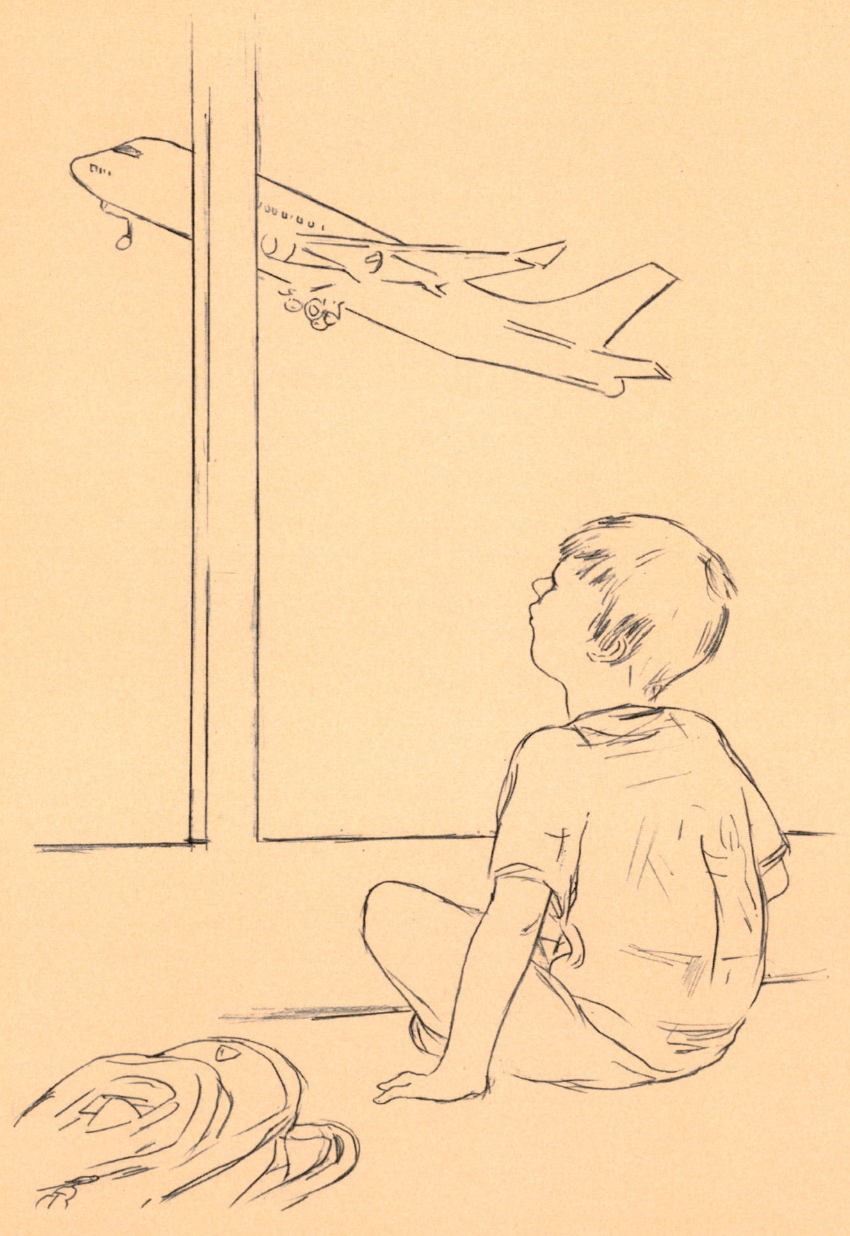

For the parents of allergic children travelling requires just a little extra planning – doesn't everything!

Car

Gone are the carefree days of just flinging everything in the boot, jumping in, taking the journey as it comes and stopping for food when you feel like it. Here are some suggestions to make car journeys easier again:

- Take a packed lunch. Do not put in any new foods – rely on those you know and trust.
- Plan your route before you leave. Decide roughly where you would like to stop to eat. You may feel more secure near to a town, rather than in the middle of nowhere.
- Make sure that there are two adrenaline auto-injectors easily accessible.
- Carry a mobile phone – with the battery fully charged and plenty of credit.

If you eat at a service station, the same precautions apply as for any restaurant (p.108). However, there are additional factors to take into consideration:

- The food is less likely to be cooked from fresh on site so staff may have a limited knowledge of ingredients and will not be able to cook something special.
- It will be hard to find a pre-packaged sandwich that does not contain butter or mayonnaise.

If you know of a fast-food or restaurant chain (p.108) that serves food your child can eat then it is probably your safest option.

Aeroplane

Most airlines cater for special dietary requirements, including allergies. It is worth telephoning your airline in advance to find out whether they are able to cater for your child.

- For milk and egg-allergic children many airlines will offer a vegan meal. However, these may contain nuts, soya or wheat.
- Before the meals are distributed on the aeroplane, those who have pre-ordered special diets will be asked to make themselves known. These dishes are clearly labelled and usually given out first.
- It is still sensible to take your own snacks as there is absolutely no guarantee that your child will want to eat what is provided.
- Be warned that if your child has multiple food allergies you may find that none of the special meals provided are suitable. In this case you may be able to take your own food on board. Check with the airline that this is okay.

Check on the Anaphylaxis Campaign website before flying for the latest guidance on procedures, warnings and flying with adrenaline auto-injectors. It also contains a detailed section on peanut allergies and flying.

Medication on flights

Always pack your child's medication as hand luggage because you may need it on the journey. Adrenaline injectors in particular should never go into the hold because the cold will damage them, so carry any spares in your hand luggage too. Should anaphylaxis occur during a flight you will be wholly dependent on the adrenaline injectors you are carrying. For this reason it is absolutely essential that you have at least two available.

Doctor's letter

Since September 2001 any injectable medication taken on board an aeroplane must be declared. A written note from your doctor stating that adrenaline injectors are to be carried with the child at all times will be required. Telephone the airline once you have the doctor's letter and they will put a message on the computer saying that you have a medical note. Without the letter you might find that your emergency kit is placed under lock and key accessible only to the flight crew. Give your GP plenty of time to write the letter. Most will be willing to do this for free; others may charge a small fee according to practice policy.

Nuts on board

Nuts are given out far less often on aeroplanes than they used to be. The few airlines that still do so are usually prepared to ban nuts for a flight if they have allergic passengers aboard. You will need to give plenty of warning by telephone and then a final check during the week before the flight. When checking in and on boarding remember to remind the crew of your requirements.

On the plane, we ask the crew to announce that there is an allergic child on board. They can ask passengers not to eat peanuts on your flight. Tom

Please remember that, even if an airline does not serve nuts on your flight, they have no control over other passengers bringing nuts on board.

Delays

Think before you go to the airport about how you will cope if the flight is delayed for a long time. Packing an extra lunch box for your allergic child is a wise precaution.

TOP TIP

Always ask for help, from strangers if necessary. Do not struggle on your own.

Ferry

As far as eating on board goes, it is much like being at a motorway service station (p.121) and taking your own food is always the most reliable option.

I pack a flask of soya milk for Thomas and then buy a small packet of cereal if we're travelling early in the morning. He's also happy to eat toast with jam (from the individual, sealed mini-containers) without butter. Deborah

I use the mini-packs of dairy-free margarine for travelling with Matthew. I buy them from our local supermarket and they're great, I always keep a couple in my handbag. Gwyneth

If you're booking with a travel agent, ask for their help. Can they contact the ferry company in advance to find out which foods they stock in their canteens? Is there a sit-down restaurant with waiters and waitresses where it will be easier to explain about the allergy? This will be an expensive option for a large family but may be worth it.

Should anaphylaxis occur during a ferry crossing you will be wholly dependent on the adrenaline auto-injectors you are carrying. For this reason it is absolutely essential that you have at least two and carry them at all times.

Trains

Trains carry a limited range of pre-packed sandwiches and pastries so it will be difficult to purchase food for allergic children. On long journeys, the easiest option is a packed lunch for the family. You can make it part of the adventure by putting the lunch in little backpacks so each child can carry their own.

Packed lunches have become the norm, and I automatically carry food in my bag wherever we're going. Sue

If your child should suffer an anaphylactic reaction on a train, ask someone to summon the guard whilst you treat your child. The guard will arrange for the train to stop at an appropriate station and for an ambulance to meet you there.

If there is no guard on the train, call 999 and explain that you need an ambulance to meet you at the next station. The ambulance staff will be able to tell you which station the ambulance can reach and an operator will stay on the telephone with you until you are picked up.

Public Transport

On all forms of public transport there is a risk that your child may pick up or touch food left behind by others – discarded peanuts, sandwich wrappers, crumbs and spilt drinks. Scanning the seats and floor and wiping surfaces nearby are sensible precautions.

Jake's story

by Dawn

Jake's allergies were not noticed straight away but feeding didn't go very smoothly from the start. Although I and the midwives and health visitors tried very hard to get the breastfeeding right, sadly there came a point where I had to use the bottle. Jake was not gaining weight; in fact, he was losing it and I was told give him a bottle or he'd end up in hospital. So I gave him his first cow's milk baby formula. We found this very hard as we were aware that children whose parents have allergies should breastfeed if possible.

Jake seemed to be doing well on the formula but at about three weeks he had colic and constipation. We tried several things to try to ease him including weaker formulas, diluted orange juice and apple juice but nothing helped. Then he developed eczema almost overnight. His skin became dry and flaky, really sore, weeping and bleeding. The GP asked about our family history, suggested we use soya formula and prescribed some ointments for the eczema. We were thrilled to find approximately 10 days later that Jake had began to feed more regularly and no longer had constipation. The eczema, however, took a lot longer to get under control.

We didn't realise the extent of Jake's allergies until we began weaning him. We had been advised by our GP to keep him free of eggs, dairy products and nuts and all was well until one day when Jake was 10 months old. We were giving him a bedtime feed and trying some new baby cereal to keep him going for a few hours, as you do. Barry gave Jake two or three spoonfuls and Jake was very sick. Wherever the vomit touched him he came up in patches of urticaria (not that we knew what it was called then). Jake was so agitated we were really quite worried. He was becoming sleepier and sleepier until quite suddenly he just collapsed into what looked like a very deep sleep. Here was this little helpless babe, raspberry-coloured and breathing very shallowly, who we couldn't wake.

I rang our surgery, got the emergency doctor's number and called that, only to be told the GP was out on a call so we'd have to wait. About 10 minutes later the GP rang and we explained as best we could what had happened. He advised us to keep trying to wake Jake and if he were to worsen we were to ring him back. He arrived over an hour later. Luckily in that time we had managed to wake Jake, but keeping him awake was far harder than waking him initially. By the time the GP arrived Jake's breathing was stronger and he was nearer a normal flesh colour.

It was the GP who thought to check the cereal packet which contained a small amount of cow's milk. It hadn't occurred to us to check the packet because at that stage we kept Jake dairy free not because we thought he was seriously allergic to it, but because we believed it made him constipated and might make his eczema worse. The GP thought that the milk may have been the cause of the reaction but he wasn't one hundred per cent sure; he also said that Jake may just have reacted badly to a virus, a chest infection. Needless to say, we were confused and concerned. It took Jake all the following day to recover; he was very sleepy and didn't want to eat. I took Jake to have skin – prick tests done privately, as we were told the NHS would do nothing until a child was over two. The tests confirmed that Jake was allergic to several things including dairy products, egg and nuts.

When Jake was finally referred to a children's allergy paediatrician, we were given the choice of the one at our local hospital or the Children's Allergy Clinic in Oxford. I chose the local one, having been reassured that the doctor was very good and worked along with the Oxford Clinic. I had just given birth to our daughter and didn't like the idea of going to Oxford on my own with two small children. The paediatrician at the local hospital turned out to be rude and arrogant, belittling our concerns, making us feel we were making a fuss about nothing. The only good thing he did was to introduce us to the hospital dietitian who turned out to be the most splendid friend in those early months.

We took Jake along to see him three times over an 18-month period. I asked about having a RAST blood test done (see p.47) because I was by now anxious to find out how allergic Jake was – and to what. The paediatrician said no, the test would prove nothing due to Jake's age. Ironically, the very next day Jake had an allergic reaction and was admitted to hospital.

While we were on the children's ward, I persuaded the doctor on duty to take the blood sample to do the RAST test. Then who should come along? None other than the paediatrician Jake had seen the previous day. He again said there was no point in doing the RAST, even though Jake's body was now fighting the very allergens he had said needed to be present for the test to work.

I wish I had been confident enough to ask to be referred to Oxford when, after our first appointment, I felt unhappy with the way the paediatrician had spoken to us and the disregard he showed for Jake's well-being.

In the beginning we were very stressed at times, either because we were not getting the help we needed or because we were overwhelmed by what was happening and the effect it had on our lives. Most people are prepared for a child to change their lives but we could not have prepared ourselves for this.

14 Trusting other people to look after your child

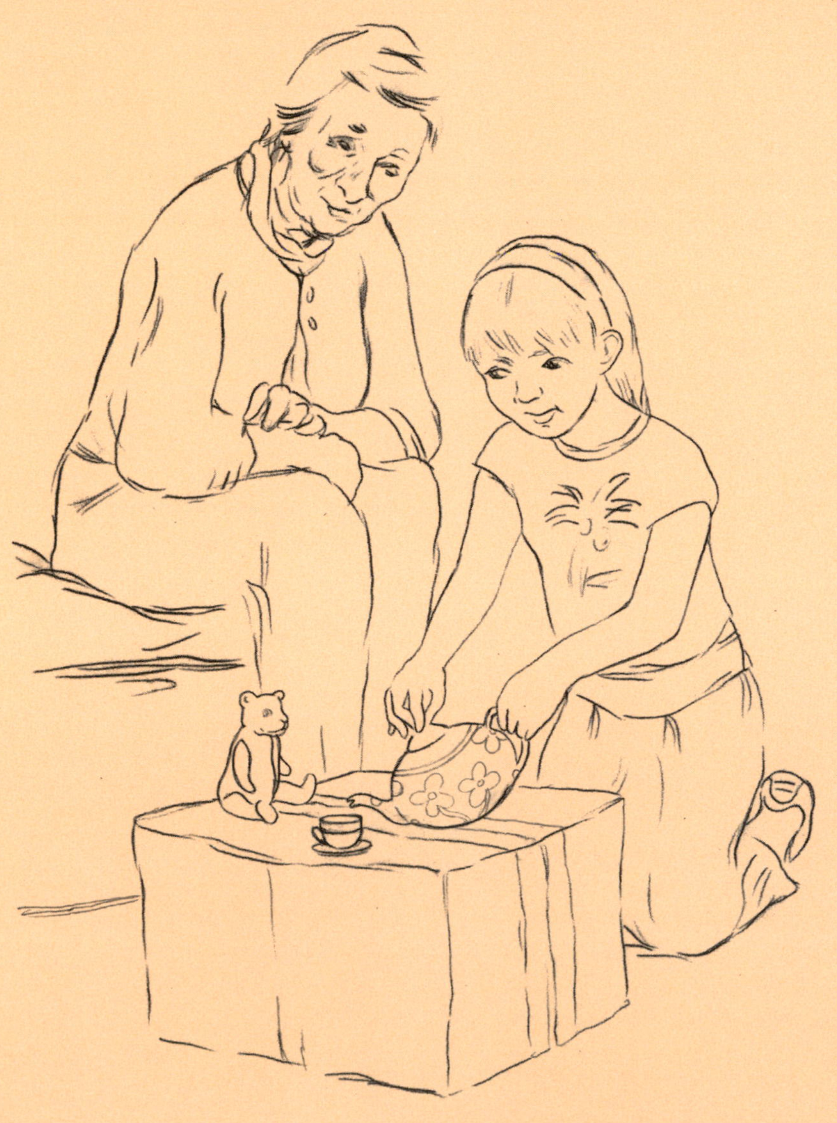

Anyone looking after a food-allergic child, whether professional childminder, nanny, au pair, babysitter, friend, grandparent or another member of the family, will need to know:

- How to prevent an allergic reaction.
- How to recognise an allergic reaction.
- How to treat an allergic reaction.

Anyone looking after an anaphylactic child, *for however brief a period*, must be shown how to use an adrenaline auto-injector and know what to do in an emergency (p.41). You are responsible for making sure that your child's medication is always easily available and that the carer knows where it is and how to use it.

In short, carers will need to be as knowledgeable about handling your child's allergy as you are. They will also need to know how to manage any asthma or eczema your child might have. This is no easy undertaking so in this section of the book we aim to help take a bit of the stress out of the process.

Childminders

Childminders are a special case because they will be taking your child into their own home. To do this safely they will need to know as much about your child's allergy as you do. Go through the relevant sections of this book with them. Above all, both you and your childminder need to feel confident that your allergic child will be safe in their care.

Professional childminders are likely to know about anaphylaxis and may even have cared for allergic children before. Don't stop assessing a potential carer because they come over as being confident, though – make sure they really are taking in what you tell them. If you are confident about the person's ability to deal with the situation, a good working partnership will be achieved. On the other hand, if you have doubts, trust your instincts and look elsewhere.

Food and drink

It is safest if you provide all meals and snacks. By preparing dishes yourself, and freezing them you can give the childminder quick and easy meals for your child. If you and your childminder agree that she will do the cooking, you must give her very clear instructions about the foods which are allowed. Devising a set weekly menu together, and a shopping list to go with it, is a good option because then you know what your child has eaten each day without lengthy discussions at pick up time. You may be lucky enough to find a childminder who is prepared to keep a record of everything your child eats. This would be helpful if you are weaning or if your child's eczema or asthma flares up later in the day. In most cases, sticking to set dishes for each day is sufficient to keep track of what has been eaten. Make sure all snacks are safe too.

Cross-contamination is a risk if other children are eating different foods, so check that the childminder knows how to minimise the dangers (separate cooking and serving utensils; sensible distance between children at table; no food swapping; and a separate flannel for your child). It goes without saying that meals should *always* be supervised by your childminder.

A special note on drinking cups and anaphylactic children

Young children will drink from any cup within reach which is potentially very dangerous for the anaphylactic child. Ask your childminder to always put cups out of the reach of other children and give them to the children either when asked for or just at set times.

Out and about with childminders

Discuss with your childminder where she can take your child for social activities such as Baby and Toddler groups. Many childminders attend local groups regularly and may not be aware of the particular difficulties that these present for allergic children. Go through the section on Playgroups (p. 103) with her. You will need to assess for yourself whether your child will be safe in these busy social environments, especially since your childminder may have other children in her care. Visiting the groups with your childminder is a good way to assess the situation, discuss pitfalls and come to a decision.

The allergy-friendly home

Childminders are required by law to put rigorous safety measures in place but you will nevertheless need to help your childminder allergy-proof her home. Some points to watch out for are:

- Can the kitchen cupboards, fridge or freezer be opened and the contents reached by your child?
- Does an open vegetable rack contain food your child should not eat?
- Can your child reach pet food either from a bowl or the packet?
- Can your child reach other children's drinking cups, bottles or snacks?
- Does the garden contain any fruit, vegetables, animals or animal foods which are unsafe for your child?

First aid

Registered childminders are trained in first aid but you will also need to teach your childminder how to recognise and treat an allergic reaction (p.41).

If Peter was to be left, then someone had to take charge of his medication and know how to use it. I found that professional childminders usually had more training than I did! Angela

Concerns about being rude

Don't worry about asking difficult questions. If you are naturally shy or feel intimidated, ask yourself whether it is really worth putting your child at risk just because you might sound rude. The childminder will understand, especially if you explain that you do not wish to cause offence but that you need to put your mind at rest.

A childminder may want to ask you the following questions:

- Can I have a list of all the foods your child can't eat?
- So what can they eat?
- What do I do if they eat something they can't have?
- I usually cook lunch for the children. Is it going to be really complicated if I have to cook separately for your child?
- Would you check the ingredients of the foods for me?
- Is it okay if I'm out and want to take the children for a meal?
- Could you please label your child's food boxes and cup so I don't get them muddled up?
- Can I take your child to toddler group?
- Do I need to take the medication everywhere with me, even if we're not eating?

Once you have had a thorough discussion covering all these points (and visited the childminder's home) you will be in a strong position to decide whether you feel confident about leaving your child in this person's care.

And don't forget...

- To hand over the adrenaline auto-injectors to the childminder.
- To keep your mobile phone switched on.
- To pick up the adrenaline auto-injectors and not leave them at the childminder's at the end of the day!

Nannies and au pairs

Many of the same procedures as for childminders apply. However, as nannies and au pairs work in your own home you will be able to monitor what they cook. Be sure that safe snacks are always available.

A language barrier may make it more difficult for au pairs (and some nannies) to understand how severe allergy can be and to grasp the practical side of caring for an allergic child. If, between you, you can translate the instructions into your au pair's own language so much the better. Again, judge for yourself how competent you feel she is and don't make unrealistic demands of her.

Remember that the code for dialling an ambulance differs from country to country so be sure your nanny or au pair knows that in the UK it is 999. Produce an emergency action plan wall chart with clear instructions on what to do should she need to treat an anaphylactic reaction. Make sure she also has a copy to carry with her when out of the house. Your nanny or au pair might like you to write down what she should say if it is necessary to dial 999. Pin a copy up by the phone.

Shopping with nannies and au pairs

If you are expecting a nanny or au pair to shop for the family we recommend that you familiarise her at home with the packaging of food you buy regularly, then shop together the first few times, and always give her a detailed shopping list including brand names. With time your nanny or au pair will become as adept at shopping as you; in the meantime give her as much help as you can. Remember how stressful you found shopping at first and be patient, especially with an au pair who may be young and struggling with a new language. Remember that reading labels will be particularly hard for her.

Babysitters

The key to successful babysitting is to only put out food for the children (and the sitter) that is completely safe. Meet him or her in advance and make sure you explain all about your child's allergy before the date. Here are some basic guidelines:

- Allow fifteen minutes before you leave to go over key points again and for your babysitter to ask any questions.
- Feed your child and if possible put them to bed before you go out.

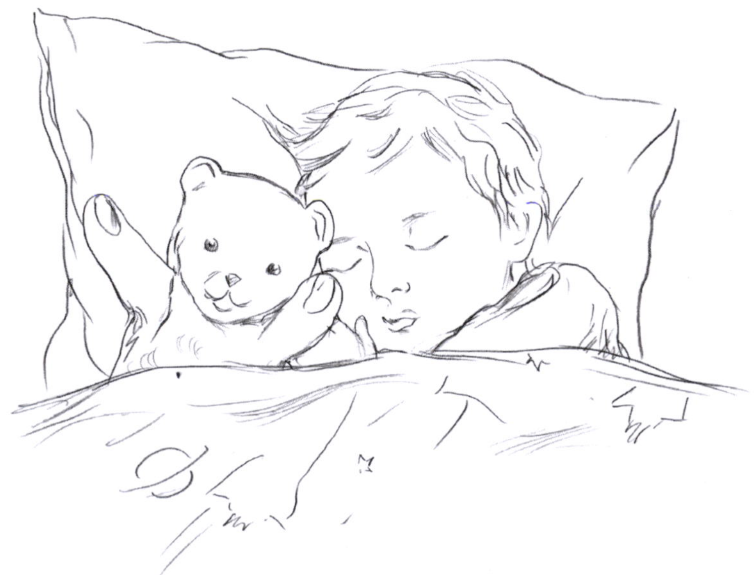

- Do not assume that your child will not wake up. Leave a bottle, a drink or a snack which the babysitter can give if needed.
- Make sure the babysitter knows to only give your child what you have left out.
- If any trace of the harmful food could cause a reaction, remind the babysitter to wash his or her hands and face before picking up your child. Leave a snack for the babysitter and ask them not to bring any of their own food into the house.
- Leave an emergency action plan alongside your child's medication in a prominent place.
- Make sure that your mobile is charged and switched on.
- Leave details by the telephone of where you are, including landline phone numbers just in case your mobile has no signal at your destination.

If you have not yet left your child in the care of a babysitter, it is easy to put off going out for an evening on the basis that it is not essential. For your own emotional well-being, however, taking time off is *extremely* important and even an hour's freedom can make you feel better: after all, your child is sleeping and doesn't need to be fed.

I think it's far more stressful to leave Katie with someone else than to have her with me. Even the most concerned people, like grandparents, make mistakes like cutting up Katie's sausage with the same knife and fork they're using to eat their fried egg with for example. Even when I leave food for her, they will inevitably give her a 'treat' which I haven't checked. Tracy

Relatives

Children usually enjoy being taken out for the day by aunts and uncles and staying with grandparents. Allergic children are no different. There may be all sorts of occasions during their childhood where your extended family will be responsible for your child's safety.

After the shock and upset of discovering Thomas had life-threatening allergies to so many things I wondered how I was going to cope when I looked after him. When Deborah is around I can check things with her but when I look after him on my own he is my responsibility and although I know exactly what to do it is still scary.

The first time I had him was the worst. I worried, 'What if one of the other grandchildren gives him something and I don't notice?' Even though I read and reread the ingredients in everything I'd still watch for the slightest reaction he might have. The thought of sticking a needle in your grandchild is horrifying even though I know it would save his life.

The first time I saw Thomas have his adrenaline during an anaphylactic fit – his screams were heartbreaking. Not only do you have to watch your grandchild suffer with all aspects of allergy, like eczema, asthma and missing out on so much, you are also watching your daughter suffering and you feel so helpless. You just want to take the pain away but you can't. Irene (Thomas' grandmother)

Relatives may have a deep emotional attachment to your child and a natural concern for their welfare which marks them out from any other carers. They will have their own fears and worries for their young relative and how much responsibility they have for your child will differ from family to family. Some relatives join the Anaphylaxis Campaign or Allergy UK to learn more about allergies. Membership of Friends of the Anaphylaxis Campaign is specifically for relatives of allergic children who wish to receive up-to-date information. Other family members will rely on you for their information – a copy of this book would be a good place to start!

I gave Matthew's grandparents allergy books for children for them to read to him. The subtle approach! Gwyneth

I love having fun with my nephews, being energetic and silly – we have a lot of laughs together and that's important to me. I'm conscious of trying to treat him like my other nephew. I try hard not to let the fear of what a slip-up could do to him to interfere with our joyful relationship. Nonetheless, there's a sense of loss for me, him having to deal with problems well beyond his years. Eve (Zac's aunt)

Suffering with hay fever myself from girlhood, I was aware that the incidence of allergy in children was steadily rising but my knowledge was vague and out-of-date. I was, for example, astounded to find that all commercially produced foodstuffs carried allergy warnings, something I had simply not noticed. I've bought the same brands for years so it never occurred to me to turn over a packet and examine the small print on the back.

Little by little I've caught up. I try to empty our own house of dangerous foodstuffs when they come to visit. I know which ice creams are egg and nut free and now only occasionally set off with Zac leaving his adrenaline behind in the house.

If there's an impromptu change of plan I am still capable of making mistakes. I recently found myself nipping off to the post office with Zac, while his medication went to the supermarket in his brother's pushchair with John (my husband). Another time, Zac and I bought 'Royal Icing Sugar' (with added dried egg-whites) by mistake, simply because I had no idea such a thing as this existed! My failure to read the packet, because I thought icing-sugar was harmless, could have proved fatal. Ingredients in commercial products do change and there is one rule only for grandparents: take nothing for granted, make no assumptions and ALWAYS read the label. Claire (Zac's grandmother)

Grandparents as childminders

It is increasingly common for grandparents to assume the role of childminder, looking after their grandchildren regularly, maybe picking them up from school every day and giving them tea or looking after them full-time while parents are at work. If the children go to their grandparents' home the same guidelines as for childminders will apply. If the grandparent comes to your home, a mixture of childminder and babysitter guidelines will apply.

One of the differences between grandparents and professional childminders is that grandparents are not usually trained in first aid. If you or your relatives feel you would benefit from first aid training, the St John Ambulance and Red Cross run courses across the country. For everyone's sake, make sure that you teach grandparents about caring for your allergic child as thoroughly as you would a professional childminder.

Making it easier for grandparents:

- Make sure they have a mobile phone, it's switched on and has plenty of credit (and they know how to use it!).
- If they are shopping and cooking for your child, give them as much information as possible (pp.80, 86) and check that they can read the tiny print of ingredients lists. Devising a menu and shopping list to go with it can be very useful.
- Make sure you are always contactable. Don't assume that because they're family they can cope with an emergency.
- Help them allergy-proof their house, especially kitchen cupboards and the fridge.
- Make sure that sweets or nuts on sideboards are put away.
- Ask that dishes of pet food are not left out (particularly for crawlers, toddlers and small children).

Allergy! What allergy? is a mind set of those of us brought up in the '50s when there weren't any allergies or so it seemed. I suffered initially from being a product of my time.

Of course I would have said I took his allergy seriously but then I'd find myself thinking, 'Just kissing him after eating an egg – come on!' I don't remember exactly what changed my mind but suddenly the thought of losing this delightful boy filled me with apprehension and guilt.

Although I well remember disinfecting the fridge and every knife and fork in the house before a visit, cooking at both houses has made me more relaxed, especially as our own diet has become almost egg free. In truth, those early months of scrutinising packets and tins made me realise just how many hidden ingredients there are in prepared foods. As a result our diets are dominated by fresh ingredients now.

There are some sticky moments still but I admire the way Zac makes light of a huge burden. I like how we work our way through the ever changing array of ice creams and lollies together, licking away at our 'mini-milks' feeling good about life.

So, have I got it now? I think so but I still go off without his adrenaline sometimes. Still learning! John (Zac's grandfather)

Staying in hospital

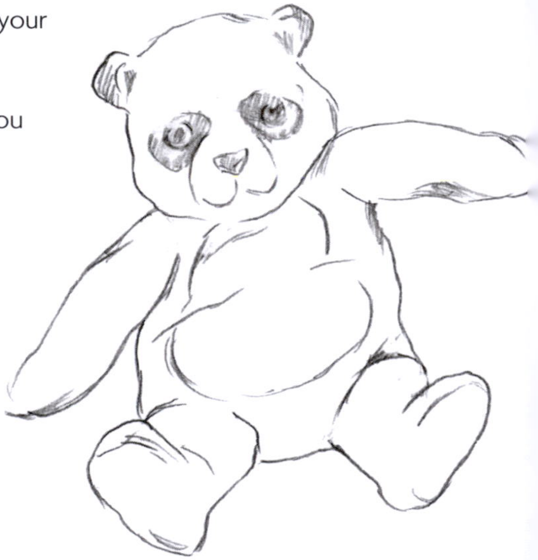

Unfortunately, there may be times when your child has to be admitted to hospital. Whatever the reason for the stay, food will inevitably be a complicating factor. You might expect that a hospital would be excellent at catering for special dietary requirements; that upon admission, the dietitian would come and discuss your child's diet so that the catering staff could choose suitable dishes from their selection, prepare them safely and deliver them to the ward clearly marked for your child. If only reality lived up to expectations.

The hospital wasn't really geared up to feeding Daisy even though she was in a children's ward. I don't think I realised how stressed I was while she was in hospital; it wasn't until afterwards I really felt awful. I didn't need that hassle. I just wanted to know she'd get the food she needed and not have to worry about it. My husband had to stay with her while I came home to get her food. I'm just glad it's all over. It was awful. Alison

Even if a dietitian is available, some hospitals do not have kitchen staff who can deal with certain allergy combinations. They have usually worked out how to safely feed diabetics, coeliacs, and patients with an allergy to nut, milk or egg but cannot cater for multiple allergies. So you may well find you need to bring in food from home.

Taking in your own food

Having to leave a very sick child in hospital in order to go home and prepare his or her food is distressing. The logistics are also difficult, especially as you want to be with your child as much as possible. Ask for help from relatives and friends, either to sit with your child or bring in suitable foods. It is unlikely that there will be anywhere to prepare food on the ward but they often have a microwave which you could use to reheat meals. Ask staff if there is a fridge where you could store your child's food. (Check that it is accessible at all times, not locked overnight for example.) Remember to put the food in a tub marked clearly with your child's name.

Staying in hospital far from home

You child could be referred to a centre of excellence many miles from home or even admitted to hospital while away on holiday. In such cases, preparing food at home will be out of the question and you would have no option but to insist that the hospital dietitian and catering staff find a solution. Find the nearest supermarket and buy supplementary foods if necessary.

The provision for allergic patients in hospital is clearly unsatisfactory and will not be changed overnight but it is worth writing to the hospital later and suggesting how it could be improved. Ask the hospital to reconsider the efforts that are made in the kitchens for both allergic children and adults. Hopefully this problem will decrease as Hospital Trusts become more allergy-aware.

15 Nursery and school

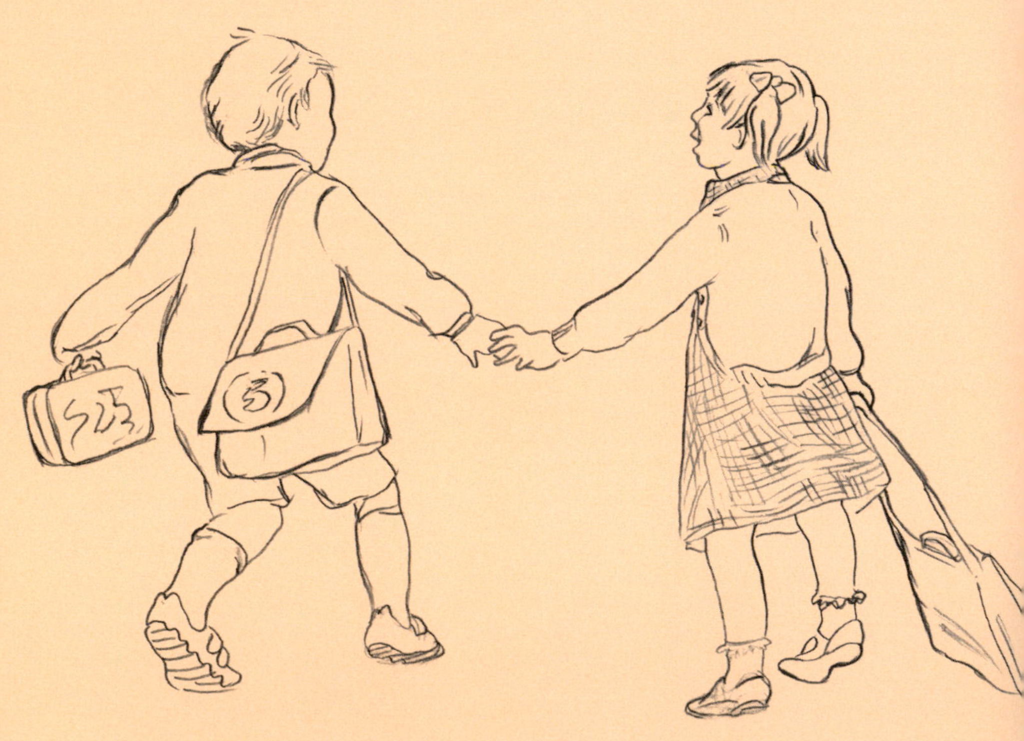

The start of nursery or school is a major event in every parent's calendar, even more so when an allergic child is leaving the safety of home for a whole morning or even a full day. Here we suggest the main factors to consider when choosing a nursery, pre-school or school.

Day nursery

Day nurseries should be allergy aware and able to make good provision for coping with your child's set of allergies. Our experience, however, is that this is not always the case. As your child could be eating up to three meals a day provided by the nursery staff you need to be very sure that they are well informed and competent.

Daisy eats what the nursery cooks and they have a list of what not to give her. I provide her breakfast and her milk. The nursery has a 'no nut' policy anyway which is the thing I know she's most allergic to, so that takes away some of the worry. Alison

Preparing for nursery

If your child is already attending nursery when his or her allergy is diagnosed, you will have to reassess the nursery with regard to allergy. The same guidelines below apply to all.

Meet the supervisor to talk over your child's allergy. If you are confident they have good allergy awareness or are willing to learn then:

- Arrange to view the nursery at meal times.
- Make an appointment to meet all the staff and tell them about your child's allergy.
- Make sure the catering staff are aware of cross-contamination issues (p.14) and know how to handle your child's food safely.
- Provide a detailed list of suitable foods or go through the catering list with the cook to make sure all your child's meals are allergy free.
- Check that the staff have been trained to use adrenaline auto-injectors; if not arrange it through your health visitor (p.19). Training should be refreshed on a yearly basis.
- Ask the nursery supervisor to put in place a three to six month review to check that the special arrangements made for your child are working.
- Agree that any new member of staff must be fully briefed by you and the supervisor before they start looking after your child.
- Read *Schools protocol for allergy* (p.140) and apply the same guidelines.
- If play activities will include food (play-dough, cooking, junk modelling, etc) discuss the dangers with staff.

An ideal nursery will:

- Appoint a dedicated carer for your child who always supervises his or her meals.
- Be willing to keep a food diary so you know what your child has eaten during the day.
- Sustain an allergy-friendly environment.

Some parents find it helpful to go along to the nursery with their child for the first day or two to ensure that the allergy procedures they have agreed with the nursery work in practice. This can be difficult if you are in full-time work but you may find you can take a day's holiday or arrange for unpaid parental leave.

Special note about milk-allergic babies and children

These children are at particular risk in nurseries because no nursery can offer a milk-free environment; not only bottles of formula but baby cereals and packets and jars of baby food containing milk and its derivatives will inevitably be present. If your child is anaphylactic to milk you may decide that the measures needed to keep him or her safe are overwhelming. Much will depend on the severity of your child's allergy and whether he or she is contact-allergic.

Pre-school

Preparing for pre-school

Children attending pre-school for a half-day session do not usually eat a meal but will be given a drink and snack mid-morning. Before your child starts at pre-school it is important that you meet the supervisor to discuss your child's allergies.

Read *Schools protocol for allergy* (p.140) and apply the same guidelines. In particular, find out what the arrangements are for snack time:

- Do the children provide their own snacks?
- Does the pre-school give water, juice or milk?
- Are the children given a biscuit or some fruit?
- Do the children sit still on chairs whilst eating or are they allowed to wander about?
- Do they wash their hands before and after eating?

It is reasonable to expect the pre-school to provide snacks that are safe for your child. Give them a list of suitable brands or suggest fruit. If you offer to buy the snacks on behalf of the pre-school, an arrangement for reimbursement is usually easy to set up.

Many pre-schools that have previously given the children milk to drink stop doing so if a milk-allergic child joins. Juice or water are good alternatives.

Finding a pre-school meant lots of ringing up and visiting places until I found one with what I considered to be the right attitude: a clean environment, lots of supervision at snack times and where the staff were willing to check foods and play stuff like play-dough or paint for ingredients that might affect Jake. Then I approached the manager to see if they would alter their usual snacks to accommodate Jake. The nursery and I agreed that it would be a lot easier and safer if all the children attending had the same snack. This means that Jake is not the odd one out. So I turn up with bag-loads of biscuits when they need them. Dawn

Play-dough

It is a good idea to check the ingredients in the play-dough that will inevitably be a part of the pre-school day. One of the assistants usually makes the play-dough at home. The basic ingredients are wheat flour, oil, bicarbonate of soda, food colouring and salt. Occasionally people still scent it with almond oil or essence. Wheat-allergic children should not be using home-made play-dough because even if they don't eat it, it will get under fingernails and small children put their fingers in their mouths.

Cooking

As part of their curriculum, pre-schools will have times when the children decorate, or even cook, cakes and biscuits. Taking part in cooking is such a positive message for food allergic children that you will, where possible, want your child to join in. Ask to be given plenty of warning about cooking sessions so that you can advise on ingredients appropriate for your child. Teachers may be grateful if you offer to buy the ingredients yourself. Wheat and eggs are likely to be the biggest problems for cookery, but there is no reason to make something that requires them at every cookery session. There are enough milk-free alternatives (i.e. dairy-free margarine or soya milk) to make baking possible for milk-allergic children. You might like to take in your own favourite recipes for them to try.

Matthew's nursery is clued up and they have always been very good. They check ingredients carefully for food play and cooking. He's never unsupervised. Gwyneth

There may be cooking days when you feel it is safer to keep your child at home. Sometimes we just have to accept that there are things our allergic children cannot do. They will be none the wiser as long as you don't make a fuss about it.

Lunch

Some pre-schools have a Lunch Club where parents can send in lunch boxes. Follow the guidelines for lunch boxes in school on p.142.

Junk modelling

Parents are often asked to bring in old boxes and tubes for junk modelling. The pre-school will need to check these for seriously allergic children.

One day all the children came out of school with junk modelling creations. Daisy's was made entirely from chocolate peanut cartons! I didn't know whether to laugh or cry really. Alison

Primary school

Schools Protocol for Allergy

Before your child starts school you will be required to put in place a set of guidelines (a protocol) with the school, your child's doctor and the local education authority (usually represented by the school nurse). In most areas you can organise this through your school nurse. If you need to organise this yourself, Allergy UK has produced a guideline document to help you. The Anaphylaxis Campaign also run a site dedicated to information for schools.

The main objectives in producing a protocol are:

- To give specific details about your child's allergy.
- To provide the staff with a step-by-step guide to looking after and treating your child.
- To ensure that members of staff have been trained to recognise an allergic reaction and respond appropriately.
- To provide a signed contract ensuring that the school will keep to protocol guidelines.
- To reassure the parents that their child will be properly looked after in school.

Some schools pin photographs of children with medical needs up in the staff room and office. Ideally the photo should be mounted on an A4 piece of card with the medical details written underneath. This ensures that all the teachers and office staff can recognise children who may require emergency treatment and at a glance remind themselves what course of action to take.

When Lorie started school we were very nervous and protective but the members of staff have been excellent. We supplied written advice on the allergies, symptoms and treatment. Laminated information sheets, including a photograph of Lorie, were posted around school to ensure teachers and pupils were aware. Lorie sees that she is special but is not picked on because of this. It is a requirement that teachers are trained to use the adrenaline auto-injector in emergency situations and we are always invited by the school nurse to attend the training. Lorie's fellow pupils and teachers treat her normally and, if anything, go out of their way to make life easier for her. Lilly

Preparing for primary school

Primary school is the first time for many parents that their child will regularly eat a meal outside the home. So how should you prepare for an allergic child starting school?

- Talk to the head teacher about your child's allergy when you go to view the school.
- As soon as a place is confirmed, talk to the head teacher about implementing the School's Protocol so that they are prepared for when your child joins.

We've approached school in the same way as nursery. Although Jake does not attend full-time school for another two terms, we are already in contact with the school with regard to Jake's allergies. Adrenaline auto-injector training and protocols are in the process of being set up. Dawn

Training staff to use adrenaline auto-injectors

In the case of an anaphylactic child, it is the school's responsibility to ensure that there is always a trained member of staff available to administer adrenaline, should it be necessary. All school staff should be given adrenaline injector training including teachers, lunchtime supervisors, classroom assistants and secretaries. This can be done by a school nurse and refreshed yearly, so suggest the school puts a reminder in the calendar. Anapen and EpiPen provide training sessions for school nurses. EpiPen provides packs to help educate and train teaching staff. Discuss training with your school nurse who can also obtain trainer pens.

Our school has been excellent with Peter and his allergies. Nearly all of the teaching staff and dinner staff have had EpiPen training and they are always careful to check with me when the class has a cookery lesson. One time the whole class made shortbread with dairy-free butter so that Peter could join in. Angela

If the school has teachers for each subject, make sure that art and science teachers in particular are included in training because foodstuffs may well be used in their classes.

Medicines at school

Wherever your child is in school, their medicines must always be easily accessible. For an anaphylactic child, the school will ask you to supply two adrenaline injectors to keep on the premises at all times.

Storing medicines at school

Each school will have a designated place for storing medication. They will need from you, a recent photograph of your child, a completed copy of the School's Protocol and your child's medications.

TOP TIP

Under *no* circumstances should medications be *locked* in a cupboard or room. They must be readily accessible to staff at all times.

Please note that it is your responsibility to keep an eye on the expiry dates of all medicines (p.43). Do not rely on the school to do this.

Medic-Alert bracelet

It would be wise to make sure that your child is wearing a Medic-Alert bracelet or pendant (see Appendix) so that the emergency services are accurately informed about the allergy, as it is unlikely that you will be there.

Playtime

Ask the school to devise an emergency procedure for the playground and make all the children aware of what they should do. For example, two long blows on the whistle to indicate that they must stand still until given further instructions will enable staff to attend to your child without the other pupils crowding round. It is surprising how understanding children can be when they are told about a problem and a situation is explained clearly to them.

Lunchtime

Most parents are happier to provide a packed lunch rather than chance the school canteen but it is your right to ask for a suitable school meal if you prefer. Once your child is old enough, involve them in discussions about what choice to make and what to eat. Much will depend on the quality of your school's meals and whether it has on-site catering or not.

Lunch box

If you opt for a packed lunch, you know that the food in the box is safe but you may also like to consider the following:

- Ask the school to send an awareness letter to the parents of children with lunch boxes explaining that your child has an allergy and how cross-contamination could affect them.
- Your child could sit at a separate table with one or two friends who will not have foods containing your child's allergens in their lunch-box (see *Allergy Buddies* p.143).
- You may be able to arrange to go in to school yourself at lunchtime for the first few days to ensure that the measures you have discussed with the staff are working.

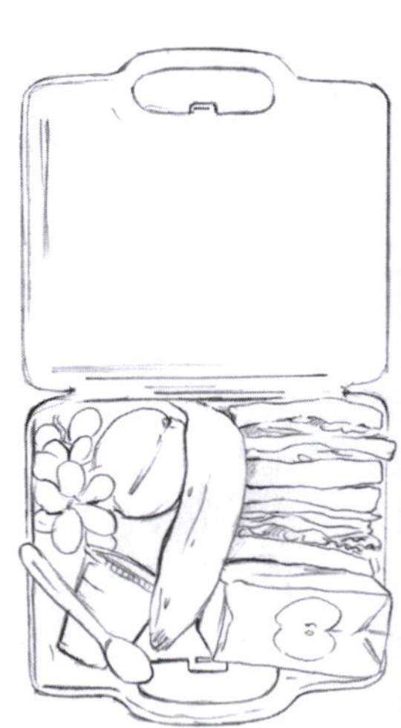

Thomas takes a packed lunch to school because I couldn't bear the stress of worrying about his meal every day. I used to worry about other children peeling the tops off their yoghurt pots and the yoghurt flicking onto Thomas' lunch without him noticing but I don't think about it any more. When Thomas was small a good friend used to make sure her son's lunch was dairy, nut and egg free so that Thomas could safely sit next to him – what a gem! Deborah

Allergy Buddies

When Zac started school, I set up a scheme we called Allergy Buddies based on inclusion and raising awareness. He has ten Buddies who bring egg-free lunch boxes and they all sit together. I provided the parents who volunteered for this scheme with recipe ideas and comprehensive information about shopping at our local stores with egg allergy in mind. All his classmates know about his allergy and it is so sweet to hear them checking that this or that is okay for Zac. I ordered Allergy Buddy stickers to go on the lunch boxes because so many children have the same box; it makes it easier for the staff. Alice

If you would like to set up a similar scheme at your school you will need to:

- Discuss the option with the class teacher, head teacher and school nurse.
- Ask the class teacher to write a letter to all parents in your child's year describing the scheme and asking for volunteers. It is important that parents or pupils do not feel pressured into joining the scheme.
- Produce a comprehensive list, with the help of the school nurse, of what is safe for Allergy Buddies to bring in their lunch boxes.
- Arrange for Allergy Buddies to sit on one table all together. Try and have a few more Buddies than places so that they can swap out to sit with other friends.
- Label Allergy Buddy lunch boxes in some way to make them easily distinguishable from other lunch boxes with the same design.
- Thank all those involved frequently! They are doing something exceptional for your child.

For full details and recipes, visit the Allergy Buddy website (Appendix).

Lunchtime supervision

A problem some parents encounter is a shortage of lunchtime supervisors which means classrooms of children eating their packed lunches unsupervised. Some head teachers attempt to solve the problems this raises for adequate care of allergic pupils by asking two responsible year six pupils to eat their lunch with them. The idea is that they are old enough to spot an allergic reaction and promptly summon help from a member of staff in a nearby classroom or staffroom. This is not a suitable solution and does not match supervision by a member of staff, qualified and willing to administer first aid and adrenaline. If the school is proposing any alternative to this fundamental level of care at what is the most dangerous time of the day for a food-allergic child, you should challenge it. Enlist the help of the school nurse and your GP if necessary.

No swapping or sharing

The danger to allergic children from swapping and sharing food at school is high. Ensure that your child knows that they must under no circumstances eat anyone else's food. Some schools adopt a strict no-swap policy for all children.

School dinners

If you would like your child to have a hot school meal during the day you should:

- Talk to canteen staff about your child's special dietary requirements.
- Give them a list of foods your child can and can't eat.
- For young children, ask to see the menu each morning and tell your child which dishes are safe for them.
- Ask that your child's meal be served first or at least enlist a dedicated member of the catering staff to ensure that his or her meal is served separately with clean utensils in order to avoid any cross-contamination.
- Accept that your child's choice of meal will be limited.
- Use the Allergy Buddy scheme (p.143). Sitting with other children forms a vital part of building friendships.

I am on the school council this year. There are 11 children who discuss problems in the school with a teacher. The committee would like to see more choice at dinner time especially for vegetarians and allergic children. We have already set up a fruit snack bar. Thomas (age 8)

Do not be afraid to check what the school intends to do at lunchtime to ensure your child is safe. Check that adequate supervision will be in place, with at least one First Aid trained member of staff present. If the children eat in a room other than their classroom their medication must be accessible.

Home dinners

If you live close to the school you may choose to take your child home at lunchtime. This is clearly the safest option but you may like to consider the following:

- Your child does need to learn how to manage his or her own allergies. School is a good place to start learning independence.
- Accommodating an allergic child during mealtimes will help to encourage the school to take its responsibilities seriously the rest of the time.

Whether you decide on a lunch box or school dinner, your child's table must be supervised by a member of staff trained to recognise and treat an allergic reaction. TOP TIP

- Your child may miss out on the fun of the playground and may find it harder to form good friendships.
- You will always have to be available at midday for an hour.

Basic safety rules for pupils:

- Hands should be washed with soap before and after meals.
- No swapping or sharing of food in school.
- Tell your child not to pick up and play with food or litter found in the playground but to tell a teacher. Playgrounds should be clean but in reality they rarely are, especially in the summer if the pupils eat their lunch outside.
- Make sure your child is supervised by staff trained in how to recognise and treat allergic reactions.

If, before your child starts, you still have serious misgivings about the school's ability to take responsibility for your allergic child then it may be time to look elsewhere for a school place. Your child's safety is paramount and a good school will understand and endorse this.

Bullying

Is your child being bullied or teased because of his or her allergies? Is he or she bullying others? Talking to your child about how friends and teachers treat him or her will help you understand what is going on. Role-play is a good way to help your child deal with situations that are worrying or people who have upset him or her. Try asking your child what other people say – starting an allergy record book together can encourage him or her to talk about it. Put in a special section for all the good things friends and teachers have said and done and another one for any bad things. Write down the times your child has dealt well with something that upset him or her. Encourage your child to decorate it with pictures or photos. Not only will it help now but you'll both enjoy looking back on it later.

You could also buy the *New Kid on the Block* DVD from the Anaphylaxis Campaign which looks at some of the issues faced by allergic children. Your child's teacher may like to show it to the class.

Fundraisers

One of the things we've found is that fundraising at school often involves food. I always have to cook special cakes and ensure that Daisy buys her own cakes back on cake sale day. She takes in her own hot dog and cake to school on hot dog day. Alison

School trips

A school trip may range from an hour at the swimming pool to a week-long field trip. Whatever the length, the teacher in charge must carry the adrenaline auto-injectors at all times. The school is responsible wherever your child goes for his or her adrenaline auto-injectors and other medication.

A day-long trip will entail a packed lunch. Lunchtime supervision of your child must not differ from the policy in place when the children are on school premises. Only one member of staff at a time should be responsible for keeping an eye on your child because if two or more share the responsibility, it is all too easy for each to assume that the other is watching.

School trips that involve overnight stays are usually introduced in the last years of school, when the pupils are 10 or 11 years old. By this age most allergic children understand well what they can and can't eat but should not have to take responsibility for choosing safe foods from a canteen.

- Talk to the catering manager at the establishment that will be feeding the children on the trip. Read the chapter on *Eating Out* (p.106) for guidance.
- Send a letter to reinforce the discussion with details of your child's allergens and what they can and can't eat.
- Provide teachers with a comprehensive list of all the ingredients that are not allowed so that they are equipped to check with the catering staff that your child's meals are safe.
- Supply a box of alternative milk, tinned or packet food your child can eat in case there is an unforeseen problem. Allergic children have been known to go without a meal because there was nothing suitable for them.
- Sometimes parents are asked to help with school trips. You might be able to volunteer if you are anxious about sending your allergic child on camp for a week in the care of others but still want him or her to go.

Invited to tea

As your child makes new friends at school, he or she will inevitably be invited back for tea. This means that you will face afresh the challenge of explaining to a stranger about your child's allergy, waiting while the mother in question takes this in and reacts to it, finding out whether she is happy to cook a safe meal and finally showing her how to use the adrenaline injector. On the one hand, you will be delighted that your child is making a new friend and on the other, you may have that sinking feeling of 'Here we go again' or 'Why is everything always so complicated for us?' Although spontaneity is not possible at first, you will gradually build up a network of friends who will safely cook and care for your child, providing many happy play-dates in the years ahead.

Hosts will need to know which foods to buy and cook. Arrange a time to demonstrate the adrenaline auto-injector – preferably at their house so that you can spot any potential hazards and discuss them at the same time.

I do make a point of telling him that he is having soya ice cream or soya yoghurt so that when he goes to a friend he knows what he has is different. I like him to feel included but emphasise the difference too. Gwyneth

Every time Thomas is invited out to tea I feel that old fear creeping back: that this might put him in danger. Deborah

You will have to accept that sometimes your child will not be invited for tea because of his or her allergy. Why not invite the friend in question to come to you instead?

Initially we felt quite stressed. We constantly had to explain to people how severe the condition was. We felt sorry for Lorie as some people would avoid inviting her for tea or to parties. We are much more relaxed now and have learnt to accept the fact that she may never grow out of the allergies. Tom

Clubs and sports

At some point your son or daughter is likely to want to join an out of school club. Food may not usually be part of their session but will certainly crop up in craft or badge activities, 'cook-out' evenings or celebrations throughout the year. Camping out is another popular club activity, so liaise with the leaders to make sure that the camp food is safe for your child. You can give the leader details of safe brands from a local supermarket or offer to do the food shopping for the club yourself. Give your child safe snacks of their own to take along.

The leaders will need to know how to recognise your child's allergy and how to treat any symptoms. Your school's nurse or health visitor can carry out adrenaline injector training for clubs.

Your child's medication must always be present and clearly labelled with his or her name. Check that there is always the facility to telephone for medical help should a problem occur.

Thomas goes to swimming lessons and Cubs. The leaders know what to do if he does have an allergic reaction but he is so much more at risk of asthma that the anaphylaxis isn't my biggest concern. He just takes his bum bag with all the medications in it that he might need. So far he hasn't needed anything during either club. Deborah

Some clubs are reluctant to take a child with severe allergies but as long as they inform their insurance company and are given clear advice there should be no problem.

16 Birthday parties

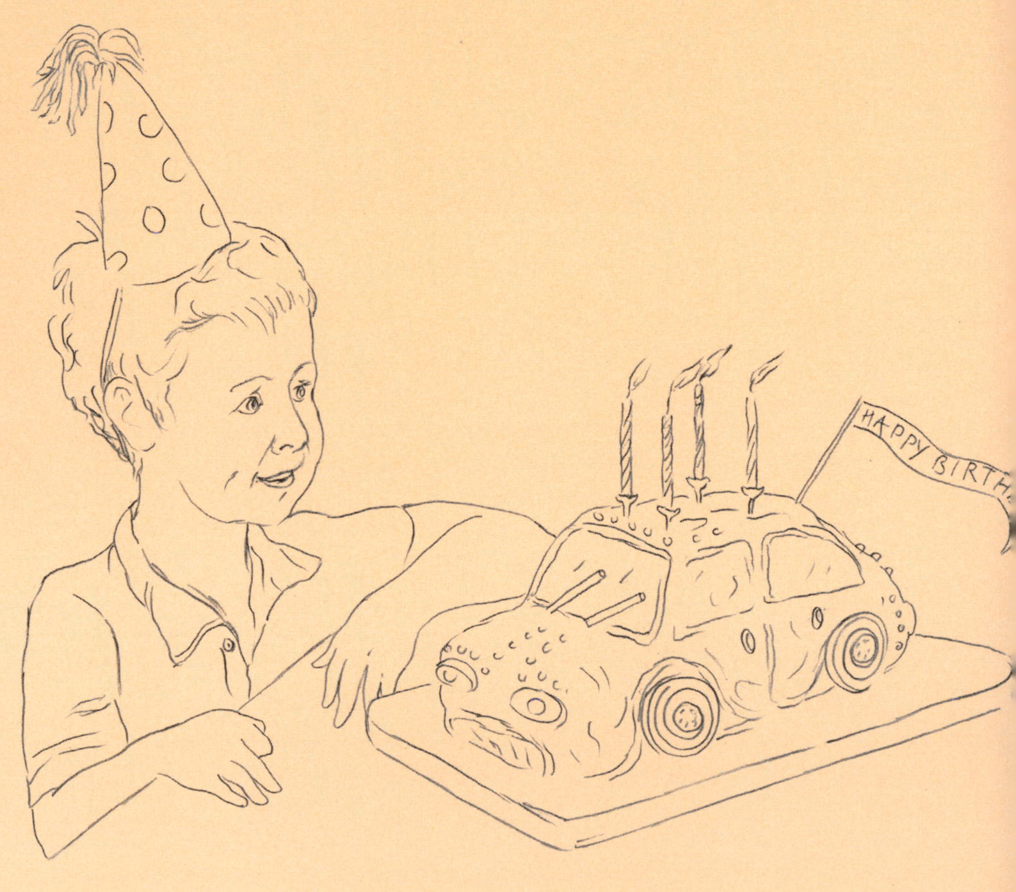

Typical party foods – birthday cake, sandwiches, burgers, biscuits, ice cream – are full of butter, wheat, nuts and eggs. Allergy-friendly parties are a tall order for people unfamiliar with allergy. In most cases, any parent who invites your allergic child to a party will be willing to make food that is allergy-friendly.

We know that it takes a leap of faith to trust someone else to cook for your allergic child, especially if you don't know them well. We hope that the options below will help you to find some solutions which work well for you and the host.

Allergy-friendly party food

When the host offers to produce only foods which your child can eat safely you will probably faint with gratitude! Once you've picked yourself up off the floor, you can compile a clear list of 'typical' children's party foods that your child is allowed (example on p.150). Find out which supermarket the host would like to use and write your list accordingly. Avoiding allergens is often just a matter of buying the right brand.

Providing recipes and advice on alternative ingredients for party food and a copy of your 'Free from...' list will make it easier to find safe options.

Providing food yourself

You can provide the host with allergy-friendly food for your child, similar to the food being served at the party. Ask them in advance what they are planning to serve and try to match it as closely as possible with the food in your child's bag, plus their favourite treat.

We've taken our own food to birthday parties and our own sweets for party games.
Angela

This option works well for very young children and some are happy for this arrangement to carry on as they get older because it means they can safely join in the fun. Older children will begin to find it upsetting or embarrassing to have special food while all their friends enjoy eating what they like and you may need to explore other options. Giving them the chance to be involved in making the decisions can help them feel more confident about the choice.

So far, we have taken a packed lunch with us to birthday parties and I try to match it to the food on offer at the party. As Jake is only four, the parties have been for close friends and family. Dawn

Supervision will be necessary because there are risks, especially with younger children who might pick up food from elsewhere on the table. Small children also like to offer things to each other and might unwittingly give your child something unsuitable. Sticky fingers are also a danger so ask if hands can be washed after tea.

Thomas: Party food list for Tesco

Thomas is allergic to all **MILK & DAIRY** products and raw or undercooked **EGG**.

He is ALLERGIC to the following ingredients:

Milk (cow, goat and sheep); Butter; Butter oil; Butter fat; Casein; Caseinates; Cheese; Cheese powder; Cream; Hydrolysed casein; Lactose; Margarine (unless it is milk-free); Milk powder; Milk solids; Non-fat solids; Whey; Whey powder; Yoghurt
Egg (raw or undercooked)

Thomas CAN eat:

Any fruit and vegetables – fresh, canned, frozen and dried
Sliced breads & rolls
Any salted or unflavoured Pop Corn
Any jam
Any jelly
Any fruit juice, squash or fizzy drinks

Frozen savouries
Lincolnshire sausages (20 pack)
Large sausage rolls (20 pack)
Party sausage rolls (50 pack)
Breaded chicken fingers (20 pack)
Oven chips
Birds Eye potato waffles or Alphabites
Birds Eye 100% beef burgers
Healthy Eating pork sausages (20 pack)

Fresh and tinned savouries
Skinless pork sausages (10 pack)
Cocktail sausages (24 pack)
Thin and Crispy Pizza Base (2 pack) – top with tomato sauce and tuna
Wafer-thin ham
Baked beans
Tomato ketchup
Princes hot dog sausages (8 pack)
Lancaster hot dog sausages (8 pack)

Biscuits
Value Digestive; Rich Tea; Bourbon; Ginger Nut; Organic Choc Chip Cookie

Cakes
Mini hot cross buns (9 pack)
Truly fruity lardy cake
Assorted jam tarts (6 or 12 pack)
Organic banana loaf
Marble cake
Angel cake
Victoria sponge mix
Kallo Organic Flapjacks

Margarine
Pure brand (500g)
Baking margarine (500g)
Soft spread margarine (500g)
Organic baking margarine (250g)
Organic sunflower spread (500g)

Ice cream
Blackcurrant sorbet
Swedish Glace – any flavour

Crisps and snacks
Ready salted crisps
Potato triangles
Potato rings
Ready salted crunchy sticks
Lightly salted Pretzels

Sweets
Jelly Tots
Fruit Pastilles
Tooty Fruities
Skittles
Haribo sweets
Starburst

Chocolate
Supercook real plain chocolate chips
Green & Black's organic dark chocolate
Ritter Sport peppermint chocolate.

ALWAYS READ THE INGREDIENTS LABEL
All foods are Tesco's own brand unless otherwise specified.

Party food boxes

Another option is to suggest that all the children have individual party food boxes. This will make it easy for your child to have his own foods, provided by either you or the host, without fuss or embarrassment.

Parties outside the home

More and more parties are taking place outside the home. If the food on the menu is suitable for your child you may decide to let him or her go, making sure a competent adult is in charge of your child, or even going along yourself. If not, then there really is no option but to decline.

There are some places we just wouldn't go, like a pizza place, as there would be nothing on the menu Matthew could eat. One of my nephews was going to have his birthday party at a Pizza Hut so I thought I'd ring up or look on the internet but I found that all the pizza bases have skimmed milk powder in them so there was literally nothing on the menu he could eat. Well I suppose he could have had salad but he doesn't like salad! So we had to blow that one out. Gwyneth

As they get older, along come the invitations to cinema, swimming, climbing wall or bowling, all followed by burgers or pizza. If you thought you were stressed before, just wait for these! The problem is that your child will want to go to all these exciting parties so badly. How can you say no? If you can be sure that the food being offered is safe and that he or she will be well supervised, then it should be possible but, if not, perhaps you can reach a compromise. You could, for example, allow him or her to go to the activity with a packed lunch or be collected before the meal.

Colour-coded plates

Don't be surprised when you come across the parent who cannot imagine how their child could possibly have a party without a certain cake, biscuit or chocolate bar. In these circumstances it is possible to have an arrangement whereby your child is told that the food on 'red' plates is fine but not to touch anything else. Clustering the 'red' plates near the allergic child will help, as will announcing the situation clearly before everyone starts eating.

This is the least safe option because cross-contamination from dropped crumbs and sticky fingers is a real worry. Also, children may well take a bite of something from one plate and then put it back on the 'red' plate by mistake. Careful supervision is vital and this option is really only suitable for children with milder allergies who are sensible enough to look carefully at what they are eating. Definitely not one for anaphylactic children, the risks are too high.

To stay or not to stay?

Young children won't mind you staying at the party so you can keep an eye on them yourself but this becomes much harder as they grow up. Don't be surprised if the host isn't too keen on the idea either; some people find it difficult having other parents around at a party. However, if you don't feel your child is safe, you may have to insist on staying to supervise or take the hard decision of turning down the invitation.

I leave Peter's medication with an adult I feel is responsible. Sometimes I hang around, at other times I wait out in the car with a good book. Angela

Birthday parties used to be a problem and we always worried Lorie would be left out because of the 'responsibility' and 'inconvenience' of keeping the food egg and nut free. However, as she has got older and made good friends, we are growing more confident about letting her go alone. She is not afraid to ask parents what the food has in it. The other parents have been very caring and supportive, always checking with us first when preparing food. Lilly

Don't feel obliged to put your child at risk out of politeness – if you're not happy with the set-up after talking to the host, insist on staying or decline. Use the opportunity to explore with your child why some situations just aren't safe. This will help him or her to make these assessments independently in the future.

TOP TIP

Once you start going to parties regularly, put together a party folder so that you can pick out the lists or information you need for the hosts quickly and easily. Slip each sheet into a plastic cover and lend it to the host. Remember to update it if necessary.

Special note for anaphylactic children

You will need to arrange a time in *the days before* the party to show the host how to use the adrenaline auto-injector (p.41). It's no good turning up twenty minutes early and thinking you'll have their attention.

Having spent time and energy making sure the food was all safe and helping the host feel less panicky about looking after Zac, I completely failed to take my own advice and show her how to use the adrenaline auto-injector in advance. As she was urging me to leave, reassuring me that everything would be fine, I had to try and show her how to use his adrenaline auto-injector, what to look for and all the rest. The colour drained from her face. I suggested I stay and her relief was obvious. I could have kicked myself. How thoughtless to put her through that after all the effort she'd made. I felt like such a fool. Alice

Remember that no matter how safe the food option you have chosen, parties get messy and your child could still accidentally come into contact with his or her allergen. Anaphylactic children must have their medication with them at all times and an adult on hand who knows how to identify an allergic reaction and administer the adrenaline.

Party bags are a big problem because they're so exciting, they're given directly to the kids and because mums tend to make them up as a job lot you often don't get a chance to vet them. It's really difficult to substitute without being obvious. You can either go one of two ways: say you can't have this, this and this but you can have this, or take along a substitute to give them. Being diplomatic about other people's birthday parties is difficult. Gwyneth

It's a fine balance between allowing your child to have a normal life, ensuring that she does not feel like the odd one out and at the same time ensuring that her health is protected. Thank goodness for adrenaline pens – it at least makes me feel that if an accident did happen then we have some sort of backup. Alison

Games involving food

Remember to ask the host if any of the party games involve food. Are they suitable for your allergic child? Are any of the prizes food or sweets?

I take a little bag of sweets with us to parties and leave them with the host, in case the entertainer gives Zac a sweet, which he can then exchange for one the host knows is safe. It puts her mind at rest, and mine.
Alice

Not invited?

The day will come when your child is excluded from a party because of his or her allergy and he or she is in tears about it. This seems a good opportunity to arrange a treat for your special child who puts up with so much.

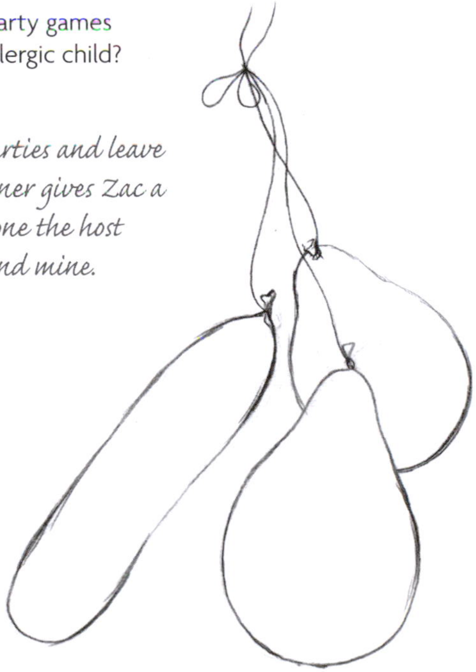

LOOKING TO THE FUTURE

17 Fear of having another allergic child

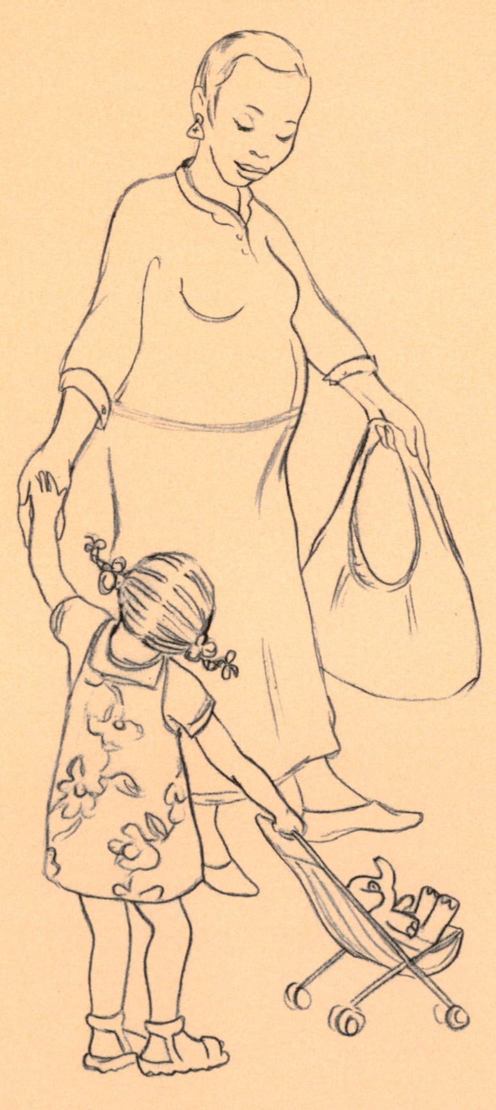

If you already have a child who is allergic to food you may be worried that your next baby will also be allergic. If you have found the experience of having an allergic child extremely stressful you may even have reservations about having another baby at all.

You may have concerns about what you should eat during pregnancy now that you know there are allergies in the family. You may be asking yourself, 'Are my children genetically predisposed to allergy? Is there anything I can do to prevent allergy? What if I eat the wrong things when I'm pregnant? If I cut things out of my diet whilst pregnant and breastfeeding is that good for me? Have I got the mental and physical energy to cope with another allergic child? What if my next child's allergies are completely different and I have to learn all over again?'

It is natural to have these fears and worries and the only practical advice we can give you is to talk them over with your child's doctor or allergist, ask for a referral to a dietitian to discuss what kind of diet you could eat during pregnancy and breastfeeding and ask your friends and family for support. Don't expect to be given any definitive answers though because there just isn't enough known yet about how allergies work, especially in the womb, to give clear guidance. The best you can do is ask for help in assessing your individual case, taking into account your family's history of allergies.

We were told that our probability of having another allergic child was 40 to 80%, but this could be any allergy – hay fever for example. We have a family history of hay fever, asthma and eczema – caused by pollens, dust-mites and cats. Both my husband and I are atopic, as are my brother and his sister. Peter's cousins both have eczema and his younger sister Alice is always itchy if she rolls around on the carpet unclothed. Our biggest worry would be having a child with a very acute allergy. However, allergies can develop at any age so you're never in the clear – you just have to get on with life. Angela

I took probiotics during my second pregnancy. I don't know if they helped but Aidan has no eczema or allergies so far. Gwyneth

We did worry about having a second allergic child. When Fay was born we were told to treat her as normal and we started her on regular formula. Eventually her milk allergy was recognised and we put her onto soya formula. Now we treat Fay exactly the same as Jake. We're waiting for tests to establish Fay's allergies before she starts nursery. Dawn

Where to seek advice:

- Your child's consultant should be able to give you specific guidance and information about the latest recommendations.
- A dietitian will help you work out a healthy, balanced diet working within the restrictions your doctor has recommended.

- Ring the Anaphylaxis Campaign Helpline for information about the latest recommendations. Research is being carried out all the time.
- Last, but not least, trust your instincts. For your own peace of mind, you'll need to feel comfortable with whatever decision you come to.

Kate Grimshaw says, 'There really is no evidence to suggest that avoiding allergenic foods during pregnancy or lactation helps prevent a child from developing allergies. In fact the most recent thinking is that the best thing to do is not to radically change how you eat. However even this advice is not substantiated by a lot of evidence. What is certain is that a well balanced diet consisting of a lots of fruit and vegetables, with fatty fish eaten twice a week will do your child no harm and may be beneficial.

'Compared to the rest of Europe, in the UK we have far more rules about what should and shouldn't be eaten during pregnancy for the health of our child, giving the general impression that tweaking our diet during pregnancy is important. In the rest of Europe they eat pâté, soft cheeses, liver and shellfish. They have the odd glass of wine and are "allowed" to take aspirin and anti-inflammatory tablets. It is interesting how different countries regard the health of mother and baby and make or do not make prescriptive guidelines accordingly.

'There really is no proven benefit from avoidance during pregnancy so try to eat what you want and not worry.'

Tips from other mothers:

- If you are restricting your diet during pregnancy or breastfeeding, find a couple of treats you can eat safely so you don't feel constantly deprived.
- Try not to make food the focus of your life during pregnancy. Eating a sensible diet and staying physically and mentally well is the most important thing.
- Every family is different so find what works for you and stick with it.

Pregnant again, I am very much living this at the moment. The things I have found hardest to work out from the advice I've been given is what is right for me. I have a philosophical approach to allergy but still find myself scared and doubtful that I've made the right choice.

There is a lot of conflicting advice on prevention of allergies, mainly because medical researchers are still working to understand what causes them and at what stage of our development an allergy can be triggered. Some doctors will advise that until more is known, there is little you can do to prevent allergy in the womb. Others advise cutting out allergenic foods whilst pregnant – a list that would frankly make your life and diet untenable.

On the one hand I feel entirely responsible for the health of the baby I'm carrying; on the other hand I'm being told by midwives and doctors how important it is to eat a balanced, healthy diet and not get stressed. Not get stressed! Who are they kidding? I am trying to limit the chances of my unborn child developing allergies by not eating any nuts and eggs in any form. With all the other usual advice about what not to eat and drink during pregnancy it can begin to feel as though giving up food altogether would be easier! Then I remind myself that I have chosen to follow this advice because deep down it makes me feel I'm doing the best I can. If this baby is allergic too, I won't be blaming myself.

What makes these decisions so hard is not knowing for sure that avoiding certain foods will make a difference. For the mother, it's a long commitment by the time you've carried the baby for nine months and then breastfed for a year or more. It certainly gives me a tiny insight into what life will be like for Zac and it is such a relief to go back to eating normally. Of course, Zac may never know what that feels like. Alice

Bearing in mind that whatever the precautions you take for your next child the prevention of allergy can never be guaranteed may help to keep the worries in perspective. You know so much about living with allergy now, that you *will* be able to cope.

We did worry about having another allergic child but our next child is free from allergies (so far). Tom

New research is emerging all the time and the advice to expectant mothers regarding allergy prevention may change. What we have written here represents current thinking at the time of publication. Talking to other mothers of allergic children, we have found a wide range of attitudes, from those who were very cautious about what they ate in subsequent pregnancies, to those who ate anything and everything. You need to do what makes most sense to you and accept that there is no proof, as yet, that what you eat affects allergy one way or the other. The right choice is the one that works for you and your family.

Katie's story

by Tracy

With my second child Katie I made a conscious decision not to introduce solids until she was 6 months old. I had done quite a lot of research and concluded that it would reduce her risk of developing food allergies.

At nine months old I decided to give Katie scrambled egg for tea one night. She loved it – every mouthful. However, about three mouthfuls from the end of the bowl I noticed that red blotches had appeared around her mouth and, on looking further, also on the backs of her hands. Then they appeared on other parts of her face that she had touched with her hands. All these red blotches then developed little raised spots, a bit like nettle rash and by now her eyes were also quite puffy. It all happened very quickly and was very alarming. I rang the doctor's surgery and was told to ring the health visitor. The health visitor was rather more concerned, said it was potentially very serious and that I should get straight to the doctor's and that they would be expecting me when I arrived.

By now (15 minutes after finishing the egg) her redness had faded a little but she still did not look a pretty sight. We were invited to sit in an empty consulting room (I'm sure that they didn't want us frightening any of their patients away!) where we were kept under observation for over one-and-a-half hours. Every 10-15 minutes either the nurse or doctor came to see how she was.

The changes to her skin during that time were amazing. Her face calmed down significantly only for her tummy to become covered in hives. They then faded as her whole trunk turned scarlet. This scarlet colour then flushed up her body down her arms and back up to her face. She also started to wheeze a little. It was very scary for me, but the doctor and nurse didn't seem very worried by it.

The doctor explained that they were watching her to see if she had difficulty breathing indicating a restriction of her airways which is potentially life threatening and would need immediate treatment, hence their constant surveillance. They were less worried about the skin reactions.

We were sent away with instructions not to give her egg again and to wait for an appointment to see the paediatric allergy specialist at the hospital. And although she sicked back up the scrambled egg a few hours later during that night, we had no after-effects whatsoever. What I find unbelievable is that throughout this entire evening of trauma for me, Katie herself was completely unfazed by it all and was her usual sunny little self, chirpy and happy.

Six weeks later we set off for our appointment at the hospital. Katie was skin-prick tested for egg and nuts. Thankfully she did not have a nut allergy and so that was one less thing to worry about.

Although we think Katie is fine with well cooked egg products (eg cakes and biscuits), because the egg problem arose early in the weaning process she hadn't really had much exposure to either. The doctor advised us to keep her diet free from all egg products for a year to prevent aggravation of the eczema and hopefully help to get rid of the allergy quicker. He also advised not to give her nut products until she is 6 or 7 years old, for fear of a nut allergy developing.

So now we have to be very careful with everything that she eats, but of course accidents can happen and so we have been prescribed with two adrenaline pens. I hope we never have to use the pens, but it is comforting to know we have them. I tried to be cautious by delaying the weaning process but to no avail. I guess the only consolation was that we were at home, during surgery hours and we could get medical attention within a few minutes. Things might have been different if her first exposure to egg had been a picnic with egg sandwiches in the middle of nowhere. It is not going to be easy scanning all foods for eggs or egg products, but I guess I should be thankful that the problem has been identified and we have a means of dealing with it should we ever need to. Hopefully, she will be one of the 97% of children who grow out of their egg allergy completely before they start school.

18 A child's allergy affects the whole family

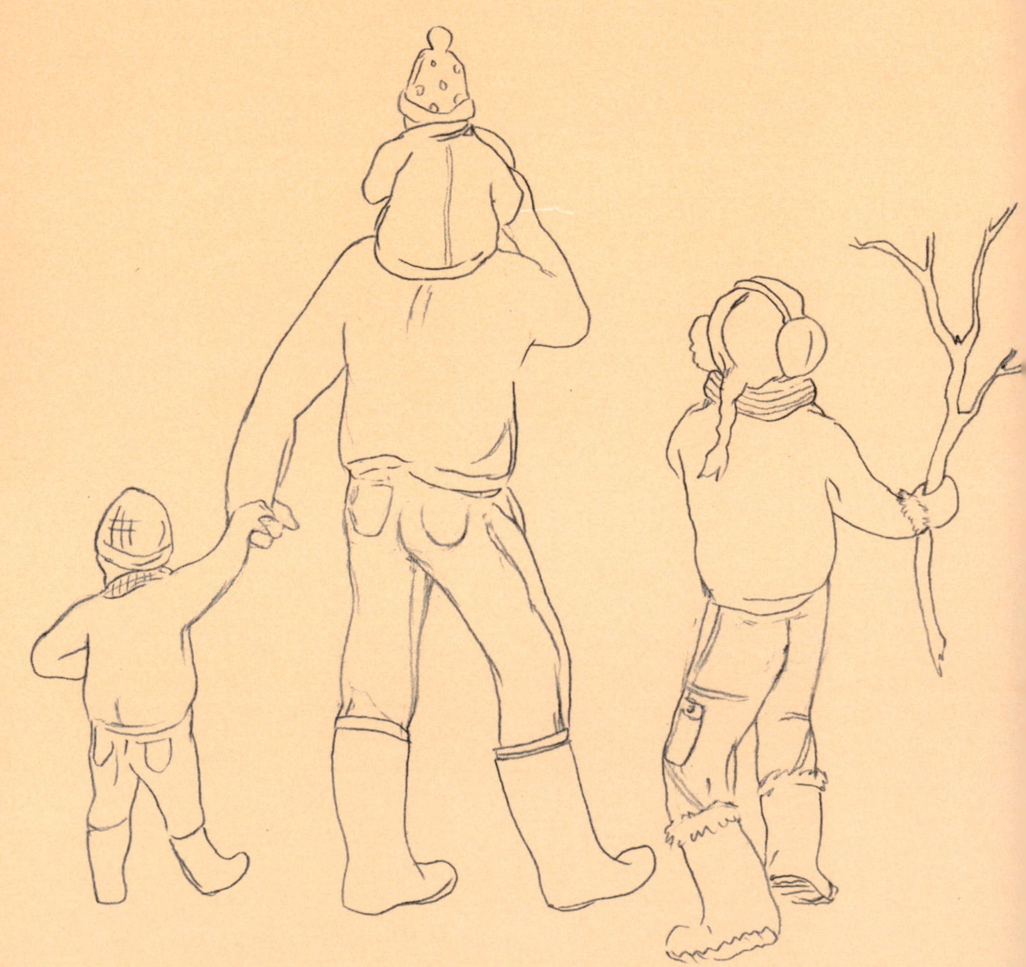

The emotional impact of a sudden and life-threatening reaction in a child can affect the whole family. The after-effects of such a frightening experience can disrupt family life, bringing out very different reactions among its members.

In most cases, these feelings can be dealt with by talking to partners, friends, siblings or the doctor, or by spending quiet time thinking it through and by concentrating on the practical tasks ahead. However, feelings of disorientation, anxiety, fear and denial may still show themselves in hostile or aggressive behaviour towards other members of the family; in shutting off emotionally; feeling unable to communicate; in refusing hugs and physical affection; in displaying unpredictable mood swings; or being consumed with feelings of guilt and responsibility for the allergic reaction.

As parents, you will be aware not only of your own emotions, but watchful for signs of stress amongst your other children and each other. Even grandparents may experience some of the same feelings. However, it is usually the mother who takes on the largest emotional burden and she can become very over-protective. It is important to understand that this is perfectly normal, necessary even, as you adjust to the new level of care that will be required.

It is also important to aim for a more balanced approach in the future, accepting that you cannot control every situation. This will happen naturally as you become used to the new situation and find your own ways of protecting your allergic child in daily life. In the long term, you will find that, as a family, you shift into new, but hopefully equally comfortable, patterns and habits. You will all start enjoying life again, unclouded by the climate of fear that seemed so characteristic of the early days. Of course the risks themselves never go away – what changes is how you approach them.

I was surprised to find myself almost in tears with anxiety when I left Zac at his friend's fifth birthday party recently. I was reminded of how nearly every social situation felt that frightening in the early days. On this occasion, I decided to stay and my instincts were right – there were foods containing egg despite the host's efforts. Later, Zac asked me why I'd come back in and I was able to explain to him how I'd had a bad feeling and felt I'd like to stay. We had a chat about coping with fears and trusting our instincts. That was good. Alice

Denial

Denial may enable you to carry on with your 'normal' family life but indicates that you may not have come to terms with the reality of allergy. You may well be putting your child's life at risk if you do not carry his or her medication or put your child in situations where he or she could be exposed to an allergen. Denial helps neither you nor your child.

Soon your child will have to make decisions about his or her safety and learn skills for independence. Growing up in denial of the allergy will not help your child to make that transition. When a child has had a life-threatening reaction to food he or she may be very fearful and anxious about another reaction or indeed any reminders of the experience. This can lead to stress and disruptive behaviour.

TOP TIP

The key to helping your child to have a normal childhood, despite allergy, is to empower him or her to decide independently which situations and foods to be wary of, how to take his or her medication, and to accept that this condition is something just to be lived with.

Taking time off

It's hard enough with children around to make time for yourself even under normal circumstances so it comes as no surprise then that parents of children needing extra care can become exhausted, depressed or ill.

If you are the **stay-at-home** parent of an allergic child you may find yourself carrying the responsibility for his or her safety every day, without a break. It is not selfish to make time for yourself – in fact it is essential for achieving a happy balance and calmer atmosphere in the home. It is also important for children and partners to see that you have needs too.

Think back to when you were out at work – did you really drive yourself that hard? Weren't there those times when you dawdled back from lunch? What about the needless cups of coffee you went out to buy, just to get a break, the time spent emailing and chatting to friends, the time spent travelling to and from work, the 'lost' memos and phone calls left unanswered, the joys of delegation? Now that you're at home, when do you give yourself a break?

Tips from stay-at-home mums:

- Go out with a friend, to the cinema, for a meal or to the pub, for example.
- Find time for some exercise.
- Ask your partner to look after the children one evening each week or fortnight.
- Book a baby-sitter or swap kids one afternoon a week with a trusted friend.
- Remind yourself that your needs are just as important as the rest of the family's.

As a **working parent**, whether part-time or full-time, you learn to 'let go' of your allergic child because you will regularly trust his or her care to others. This can be a very stressful process and cause ongoing, below-the-surface anxiety. Be aware of the pressures you are under and try to find ways to de-stress.

Working and managing childcare is a monumental juggling act, even for the working parent without allergy to consider. You will need time out to recharge, Make sure your boss and colleagues know about the extra pressures you face – don't be afraid to be honest.

Finding time to cook and having the right food in the house on the right days can be a challenge too. Rushing in from work and throwing something together for the kids' supper is hard enough without allergy to consider. Preparing and freezing meals in advance can help, as can ordering a weekly shop online which can be done when you're not in a rush.

Tips from working mums:

- Keeping a list on the fridge of favourite 'always eat it and always have it in the cupboard' meals.
- Making a weekly menu and sticking to it.
- Liaising with childminders at the start of the week to make sure your child is not going to be having the same meals for lunch and tea.
- Always having a batch of fresh veggie soup in the fridge for that ready-made vegetable boost.

Above all, go easy on yourself. Some days may be better nutritionally than others but as long as it's safe and over the week balances out well, you're doing okay. We give ourselves a hard time about food and nutrition because our allergic children are already on restricted diets. Remembering that some children refuse to eat anything but jam sandwiches and apples but still turn into fine, healthy adults can help. We cannot stress strongly enough how important it is that you take some time out just for yourself. This may *seem* impossible but it isn't.

Let other people help

Other people may take a different approach to keeping your child safe but that doesn't mean they can't do it as well as you. Try not to be too picky about *how* other people do things.

I have yet to see my husband choose even so much as a matching pair of socks for our children, but what does it matter? When they go out he always remembers to take the adrenaline and brings the children back safe, muddy and happy. The main thing is that they're off to do something that doesn't include me, and doing it their way. Alice

Don't blame yourself

You may have done everything in your power to try and prevent allergies developing only to find that they still appear. This can be heartbreaking but don't let that disappointment consume the years ahead. It is not your fault. You are not to blame. It's as simple as that.

Above all, children need the love of their parents and the security that love provides so put your energies into giving them a happy, fulfilling childhood despite their allergies. You should be reassured to know that your child's allergies might have been a lot worse had you not made the efforts you did.

TOP TIP

Try to remember that it's the hours between meals that matter.

Siblings' needs

Siblings who have themselves been frightened by seeing an allergic reaction in a brother or sister may feel that they cannot demand your attention but may very much need it. The emotional impact can extend outside the home, too. For example, children at the same school as their allergic sibling may carry a particular burden, feeling responsible or anxious for them. Watch out for signs that food is becoming a source of anxiety for siblings or being used as a means of demanding attention. Finding time and ways to let them talk about these strong feelings can be very helpful. You may like to read *How to talk so kids will listen and listen so kids will talk.*

It is easy to understand how resentment can build up if children are always denied foods they might like but which are unsuitable for their allergic sibling, or think that their allergic brother or sister is getting special attention.

I get annoyed when Thomas says he doesn't like something and is allowed to have something else but when I say I don't like something Mum makes me eat it.
Thomas' sister, Rachel (aged 12)

Watch out too for siblings eating foods they are not allowed in secret. If they are keeping food in their bedrooms there is a risk that younger siblings might find and eat it. So make sure you talk openly with your non-allergic children about how they might include 'unsafe' foods safely into their diet. If they're not allowed to bring food into the house, let them have whatever they want when you're all out together.

What really bugs me is when I ask if I can have something from the cupboard and Mum says, 'No, that's for Thomas.' But there's nothing in the cupboard for me is there? Thomas' sister, Rachel (aged 12)

Don't be blind to your allergic child taunting siblings about getting special treatment. This is normal to some degree. After all, they are so often on the receiving end of not being allowed what everyone else is having. However, allergic children need to be considerate of other people's feelings too.

Emotional support and help

If you feel that either you or other members of your family are struggling to come to terms with the impact of allergy, don't struggle alone. You can ask your doctor to refer you to a counsellor or psychotherapist or try a stress management course, for example. You may find your religion a source of strength, or benefit from joining a local allergy support group. The Anaphylaxis Campaign run support groups all over the country – contact them for more information or to set one up in your area.

Fears for the teenage years

Concerns amongst parents about their allergic children's future are common. Whilst our children are young their allergy is our responsibility and their care is in our hands or the hands of those we trust. As our children grow up, they increasingly take on more of the care for themselves. Some of the most frequent questions parents ask include: When should my child carry their own medication? When should my child learn how to use adrenaline auto-injectors? When should we teach their friends to use the adrenaline auto-injectors? Will they be able to go out with their friends without an adult? Will they be responsible enough about their allergy and medication? Will they take chances with their allergy?

Sophie, now 12, is becoming much less paranoid about her allergy as she gets older, perhaps due to increased confidence that she would be able to inject herself should the need arise. Also, her older half-brother has just got engaged to a lovely girl who also has an allergy to nuts and Sophie quite likes the fact that they have something in common! Jackie

The Anaphylaxis Campaign has responded to anxieties surrounding increasing independence by producing a free booklet called *Letting Go* which shows parents how to educate their children from a young age to manage their allergies. They also runs workshops for teenagers with anaphylaxis which are very popular. The purpose of the workshops is for young people to meet others who are food-allergic, to learn more about allergy and to share their experiences and worries. *Info for Young Adults* on their website is an informative page for older teenagers which includes movie clips showing what the symptoms of anaphylaxis look like and how to treat allergic reactions. Parents with allergic children of any age should take a look too.

15-year-old Daisy told us how having a nut allergy affects her life as a teenager. 'I never think of myself as having a nut allergy when I'm at home. I can eat everything in the fridge and anything cooked for me is safe. It's only when I'm out that I become aware of my allergy.

'I find myself making excuses about why I won't be eating with my friends or telling them I've already had dinner to avoid hurting feelings or people thinking I'm different or just being fussy.

'I find it particularly hard to explain to boys and large groups why I can't eat something and I am often surprised by the reaction I get. People tend to ask me questions about how I found out and what I can't eat. They take an interest in my adrenaline pen and are eager to find out how to use it on me if I needed it.

'Some of my friends are very careful – they wash their hands if they have eaten nuts, they scan every item of food and make me feel at ease about eating with them. But there are others who say things like, 'There are no nuts in plain biscuits' despite the warning and who think I'm strange when I choose to go to a restaurant with friends and not eat. I would rather be a part of social events than stay at home so I sit there with a large glass of coke watching everyone else eat.

'People struggle to understand that even the smell can trigger a reaction. Once I was at a party and didn't notice a bowl of Brazil nuts were spilled and crushed on the floor. The smell and maybe slight touch of them made me very ill and the bad reaction I had wasn't even related to something I'd eaten.

'When you're a child your parents are responsible for talking and warning other parents about your allergy. But as a teenager you have to do it yourself. New friends are often the hardest to tell because as a teenager you are always wanting to fit in.

'You shouldn't pretend you don't have an allergy because like many things it's something you have to deal with and there are so many ways you can get round things that exclude you. Your real friends won't think you're being fussy, they will just want to understand and help.'

Growing up and going strong

No doubt the greatest wish of every parent reading this book is that their child will one day grow out of his or her allergy. If it happens, it is an exciting time for allergy families but it can also be worrying. You doubt it can be true, and you may be reluctant to let your child eat the food you've all been avoiding for so long. No wonder! The doctor will usually advise that your child starts to eat it on a regular basis. Gradually, he or she will become accustomed to it. You will begin to relax, your fears will subside and before long, anaphylaxis will be a distant memory.

When Thomas was 11 we went for a milk challenge following an encouraging skin-prick test. I dreaded the same disappointment as last time and hardly dared hope it might be a success. I convinced myself he would react and wondered why we were even bothering. After the second stage of 5ml Thomas complained of a sore throat. I thought that was it but he had a drink of water and felt better. He continued the challenge and managed to drink the increasing quantities of milk without reaction. I can't begin to describe the way I felt. There was no reaction at any stage. After all those years it is still hard to believe.

We introduced milk carefully and slowly into his diet and he is absolutely fine. He much prefers soya milk and still has it but the complete change of life is unbelievable. No more adrenaline, no more checking ingredients, no more feelings of disappointment for him. I watched him joining in with all the other children around a chocolate fountain at a wedding recently and was filled with joy at how far he'd come. Don't give up hope – that could be your child one day. Deborah

When I was 10 I thought I probably wouldn't grow out of my milk allergy. When I had the milk challenge I was amazed to find out that I was allowed to have milk. It has completely changed my life. I can go into the shops or to a party and not bother having to look at labels to check what I can have it. I love most of the foods I can have now as well, especially chocolate! Thomas

A final word

No matter how well we manage our children's allergies and help them on their way to looking after themselves with confidence, deep down we'd all like a cure, to be rid of the daily threat to their lives. So we thought it might be appropriate to end by asking what the medical profession sees in the future for food allergy.

While at the moment we cannot cure allergy, research now has reached the stage where I think we can be very optimistic about the potential for having dramatic new ways of treating problems in the future. I think we can look forward to a time when there will be treatments which will change the whole perspective for a food allergic child. To be realistic, this is probably five to ten years into the future but at least someone with a newly diagnosed young child with allergy can expect that there will be some definitive treatments before the apron strings are cut.
Professor John O. Warner

We hope this book has been helpful to you and that you in turn can now offer help to others.

Good luck.

Alice and Deborah

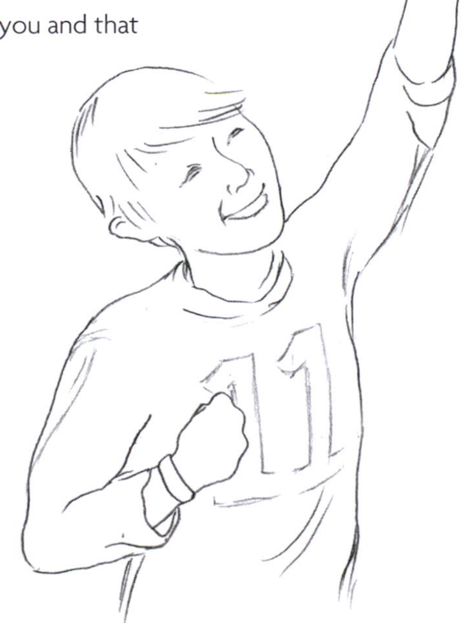

Contributors

Alice and **Martin**: Zac is allergic to eggs, cats and housedust. He was allergic to nuts. He first reacted at 7 months to eggs. He had eczema as a young child but is fine now. He has a younger brother Theo who has mild eczema.

Alison: Daisy is allergic to dairy products, eggs and nuts. She first reacted at 3 months, then to peanuts at 20 months old. She also has eczema. She has a younger brother, Alex, who is allergic to legumes.

Angela: Peter is allergic to eggs and dairy products.

Amanda: Max is allergic to peanuts.

Daisy: Daisy is allergic to nuts and peanuts.

Dawn and **Barry**: Jake is allergic to eggs, dairy products, nuts, cats, dogs, dustmite, mould, wool, bee's venom and pollens. He was ill from birth and he had his first anaphylactic reaction at 10 months. He had bad eczema as a child. He also has asthma. He has a younger sister Fay who is also allergic to dairy products and eggs.

Deborah and **Duncan**: Thomas was allergic to dairy products, soya, eggs, honey and nuts. He is still allergic to animal dander, horses, feathers, mould, dustmite and grass. He was ill from birth and had his first anaphylactic reaction at 15 months. He had severe eczema as a young child. He still has bad asthma. He has two older sisters, Rachel, Sarah (who has bad eczema and mild asthma) and a younger sister Isabel.

Gwyneth: Matthew is allergic to dairy products, eggs, wheat and nuts. He had severe eczema as a baby and young child. He has a younger brother Aidan who is not allergic.

Jackie: Sophie is allergic to peanuts but is advised to avoid all nuts. She had her first reaction after ingesting peanut butter at 8 months old. Much to Jackie's surprise, she has joined her daughter in carrying adrenaline after a very severe reaction to penicillin at the age of 41.

Sue and **Paul**: Harvey is allergic to eggs and dairy products and has bad eczema. He first reacted at 7 months to egg.

Tom and **Lilly**: Laurie is allergic to eggs, peanuts, legumes, grass, latex, cats and dogs. She first reacted at 6 months old. She has a younger sister Natalia who has mild asthma.

Tracy: Katie was allergic to eggs. She first reacted at 9 months, has mild eczema and an older brother who has eczema and a high intolerance to all artificial additives.

Thanks also to all those who contributed anonymously, your input was immensely useful.

Interviews were carried out between 2003 and 2005 and all followed up in February 2007. Ages are accurate at the time of first publication in 2007.

Appendix

Listed here are details for the organisations, companies, websites, shops and books referred to in our book. Please bear in mind that details may change, so we apologise in advance if you have any difficulties.

Allergy Charities

Allergy UK
Helpline: 01322 619898
www.allergyuk.org
3 White Oak Square, Swanley,
Kent BR8 7AG

Anaphylaxis Campaign
Helpline: 01252 542029
www.anaphylaxis.org.uk
PO Box 275, Farnborough,
Hampshire GU14 6SX

Other useful websites

www.allergyaction.org
Action Against Allergy has a page of useful expressions in several languages.

www.allergybuddies.org.uk
Allergy Buddies is a scheme for school lunches.

www.allergyfacts.org.au: Australian site.

www.allergyinschools.co.uk: designed specifically for schools and pre-schools by the Anaphylaxis Campaign. Includes a sample school protocol to download.

www.anaphylaxis.org: Canadian site.

www.insectstings.co.uk: personal accounts and information on insect stings.

Books

The Allergy Bible by Linda Gamlin, ISBN: 978-1844001729

The Complete Guide to Food Allergy and Intolerance by Professor Jonathan Brostoff & Linda Gamlin, ISBN: 978-0747534303

Food Allergies – enjoying life with a severe food allergy by Tanya Wright, ISBN: 185959039X or second edition: 978-1859591468

Allergies at Your Fingertips by Dr Joanne Clough, ISBN: 978-1872362526

Bakin' Without Eggs: Delicious Egg-Free Dessert Recipes from the Heart and Kitchen of a Food-Allergic Family by Rosemarie Emro, ISBN: 0312206356

How to talk so kids will listen and listen so kids will talk by Adele Faber and Elaine Mazlish, ISBN: 978-1853407055

Breastfeeding

La Leche League:
24 hour Helpline: 0845 120 2918

National Childbirth Trust (NCT):
Helpline: 0870 444 8708

Home help

Home Start: 08000 686368
www.home-start.org.uk

Medical

Anapen: www.anapen.co.uk
For trainer pens, ask your doctor to order one for you or by contacting: Lincoln Medical Ltd, 13 Boathouse Meadow Business Park, Cherry Orchard Lane, Churchfields, Salisbury SP2 7LD.

EpiPen: www.epipen.co.uk
You can purchase a trainer pen or Lifeline Patient Training Pack via the website where you will need to enter a valid EpiPen expiry date to purchase the training devices or by contacting: ALK Abelló, 1 Tealgate, Hungerford, Berkshire RG17 0YT

Medic Alert: 020 7833 3034
www.medicalert.org.uk
membership@medicalert.org.uk
The Medic Alert Foundation, 1 Bridge Wharf, 156 Caledonian Road, London N1 9UU

NHS allergy clinics: to find your nearest clinic look on www.bsaci.org or call the Allergy UK Helpline

NHS Direct: 0845 4647

Free From… lists

Asda: www.asda.co.uk: 0500 100055

Co-op: www.coop.co.uk: 01706 202020

Iceland: www.iceland.co.uk: 01244 842842

Marks and Spencer:
www.marksandspencer.com:
0845 3021234

Morrisons: www.morrisons.co.uk:
0845 6115000

Sainsbury's: www.sainsburys.co.uk:
0800 636262

Tesco: www.tesco.com: 0845 7225533

Waitrose: www.waitrose.com:
0800 188884

On-line food shops

www.goodnessdirect.co.uk
www.kinnerton.com

Stockists of kit for allergy sufferers

Kidsaware: 0870 2202452
www.kidsaware.co.uk

Medicare Plus: 01737 226384
www.medicareplus.co.uk

YellowCross: 01252 820321
www.yellowcross.co.uk

Travel insurance

The British Insurance Brokers Association:
0901 814 0015: www.biba.org.uk

European Health Insurance Card (EHIC):
www.dh.gov.uk/travellers

References

1 Allergy UK

2 Anaphylaxis Campaign

3 Sampson HA, Mendelson L, Rosen JP. Fatal and near fatal anaphylactic reactions to food in children and adolescents. New England Journal of Medicine 1992;327:380-4.

4 'Poorly managed asthma' is the phrase used by medical professionals to describe asthma that has not been treated with the appropriate medication. This phrase can sound a bit alarming, like so much medical terminology.

5 The most recent Department of Health recommendation states that: 'Breast-feeding is the best form of nutrition for infants. Exclusive breast-feeding is recommended for the first six months (26 weeks) of an infant's life as it provides all the nutrients a baby needs.' This was based on the conclusions of research carried out by the World Health Organisation (WHO) called the Global Strategy for Infant and Young Child Feeding: the optimal duration of exclusive breast-feeding published in May 2001 which recommends 'exclusive breast-feeding for six months, with the introduction of complementary foods and continued breast-feeding thereafter.'

6 Department of Health. Chief Medical Officer Update 37. 2004

7 Concise Oxford Dictionary

8 Department of Health recommendations.

9 Department of Health. Chief Medical Officer Update 37. 2004

10 In children the most common allergens are cow's milk, eggs, peanuts, tree nuts (almonds, hazelnuts, walnuts, cashews, pecans, Brazils, pistachios, macadamia nuts and Queensland nuts), fish, shellfish, soya and wheat which make up 98% of all childhood allergens.

11 Cereals containing gluten (i.e. wheat, rye, barley, oats, spelt, kamut or their hybridised strains). Crustaceans (i.e. crab, lobster, crayfish, shrimp, prawn) Eggs. Fish. Peanuts. Soybeans. Tree nuts (almonds, hazelnuts, walnuts, cashews, pecans, Brazils, pistachios, macadamia nuts and Queensland nuts). Celery and celeriac. Mustard. Sesame seeds. Sulphites at concentrations of over ten parts per million. Milk (including lactose). Lupin. Molluscs (oysters, clams, mussels, squid, abalone, octopus and snail).

12 Professor John O. Warner MD FRCPCH, Professor of Paediatrics Imperial College, St Mary's Campus, London.

13 Allergy UK

Index